Bone Health in Children

Bone
Health in
Children

Steven A. Abrams and Keli M. Hawthorne

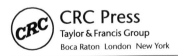

CRC Press
Taylor & Francis Group
Boca Raton   London   New York

CRC Press is an imprint of the
Taylor & Francis Group, an **informa** business

CRC Press
Taylor & Francis Group
6000 Broken Sound Parkway NW, Suite 300
Boca Raton, FL 33487-2742

First issued in paperback 2019

© 2012 by Taylor & Francis Group, LLC
CRC Press is an imprint of Taylor & Francis Group, an Informa business

No claim to original U.S. Government works

ISBN-13: 978-1-4398-4926-2 (hbk)
ISBN-13: 978-0-367-38162-2 (pbk)

Library of Congress Cataloging-in-Publication Data

Abrams, Steven A.
    Bone health in children / Steven A. Abrams, Keli M. Hawthorne.
        p. cm.
    Includes bibliographical references and index.
    ISBN 978-1-4398-4926-2 (hardback)
        1. Osteoporosis in children--Prevention. 2. Bones--Growth. 3. Nutrition. I. Hawthorne, Keli M. II. Title.

RJ482.O45A27 2012
618.92'716--dc23

2012000489

**Visit the Taylor & Francis Web site at
http://www.tolorandfrancis.com**

**and the CRC Press Web site at
http://www.crcpress.com**

Dedication

This book is dedicated to our parents, Lee and Kate Hawthorne, and Bernard Abrams, of blessed memory, who are no longer here to read this book, but who supported our education, and would have been thrilled to see that we continue to educate others.

Contents

Acknowledgments

Dr. Abrams would like to acknowledge his wife, Judith, and their children, Michael, Ruth, and Hannah, for their support and encouragement.

We would like to acknowledge the following persons for their assistance in preparing the book: Christine Keith, for assistance with the figures and tables and text review; Rabbi Judith Z. Abrams, Ph.D., for providing ancient history material; and Holly Dlouhy, M.S., R.D., L.D., Jessica Iselin, M.S., R.D., L.D., Lejuana Himes, and Amy Hair, M.D., for reviewing the text. We would also like to acknowledge the editors and staff at Taylor & Francis, Randy Brehm, Amy Blalock, Kari Budyk, and Linda Leggio for their assistance.

About the Authors

As researchers and caregivers, we have our own unique backgrounds in the field of bone health. We would like to start by describing our background and indicating any potential biases to you. We will try to fairly present our discussions, but readers should know with whom we have consulted in the near past or at the present time.

Steven A. Abrams, M.D., was a member of the Institute of Medicine panel in 1997 that established the *Dietary Reference Intakes for Calcium, Phosphorus, Magnesium, Vitamin D, and Fluoride* (The National Academy Press, 1997). He then reprised his role in the subsequent 2011 Committee to Review *Dietary Reference Intakes for Calcium and Vitamin D* (The National Academies Press, 2011). Dr. Abrams was also a member of the original 1997 Institute of Medicine panel establishing guidelines for upper limits of nutrient intakes and a separate Institute of Medicine panel in 2003 concerned with food labels and food fortification. He has been a member of the Committee on Nutrition at the American Academy of Nutrition since 2009, and he is an associate editor of the *American Journal of Clinical Nutrition*. None of the opinions in this book should be attributed to any of these groups, except as specifically noted.

Dr. Abrams is a Professor of Pediatrics at Baylor College of Medicine. He is a board certified pediatrician and a neonatologist. He practices clinical neonatology in Houston, Texas. Dr. Abrams and his research team have conducted research into bone health for over 20 years and published more than 200 peer-reviewed articles related to pediatric nutrition, most of these related to bone health. His son drank much more milk than either of his two daughters when they were growing up. His son still does, but fortunately, all three drink milk now and prefer fat-free unflavored milk. Dr. Abrams does not have a pet iguana, nor do his children, and he is fairly unconcerned about the vitamin D requirements of iguanas (Laing et al. 2001), although he has recently been concerned about too much iron in zoo bats (Lavin, Chen, and Abrams 2010).

Dr. Abrams has served on the medical advisory board for MilkPep, the Milk Processors Education Program, for several years. He does not have other financial connections to the dairy industry. Over the past 20 years, Dr. Abrams has conducted research funded by several companies who produce products related to bone health, but he has no current or recent funding in this field.

Keli M. Hawthorne, M.S., R.D., L.D., was raised in *Cowtown*, (Fort Worth, Texas) and her grandfather woke up at 4 A.M. every day to milk her favorite cow, *Zip*. Hawthorne is a registered dietitian working in nutrition research at Baylor College of Medicine in Houston, and she is a practicing clinical dietitian at Texas Children's Hospital. She has lectured on behalf of the cattle industry and the dairy industry in the past. She drank milk every night at dinner as a child and prefers chocolate milk (especially since it reminds her of her mother who drank a tall glass of chocolate milk every night before bed). Hawthorne spends her spare time swing dancing and would like to think that drinking milk while growing up helped her avoid breaking bones as a current Lindy Hop swing dancer.

Introduction

Parents and caregivers have many concerns about their children's physical and emotional well-being when they are trying to raise healthy children. Parental concern for the potential development of osteoporosis when their children become elderly is probably not a priority during childhood. Yet, just as we now understand that heart disease and diabetes are among a whole host of *adult* diseases that have their origins in childhood, we recognize that this is also true for bone health. Maintaining bone health in childhood affects our bodies both during childhood and later in life. Furthermore, establishing healthy eating patterns that will prevent osteoporosis and optimize bone health contributes to overall good nutrition; and therefore, should be, a lifelong goal.

Our intent in this book is to explore the recent decades of research and public commentary, as well as the mythology about bone health in children. We will address the components of bone, such as calcium, phosphorus, and other minerals. A discussion on the factors that affect these components, including vitamin D and exercise, are provided as we try to separate some of the myths from the realities. At times, we will expand our discussion beyond bone issues to consider interrelated issues in pediatric nutrition. Bones are connected to the rest of the body; therefore, what children eat is not defined by just one organ system. We believe it is inappropriate to feed children based on one organ system, whether it is the heart, the bones, or even the brain. There are always choices to be made about diet, and any dietary plan must consider what is known about how foods affect each of these organ systems.

Our aim is to clarify the endless, often confusing, and somewhat contradictory nature of the scientific literature geared toward those interested in bone health including doctors, nurses, registered dietitians, and families. Why are limited and often negative studies portrayed so positively? What does it mean to identify *covariates*? Covariates are factors that may interfere with a clear understanding of research study results that relate two things to each other. These factors may also help to clarify relationships between variables such as body weight and bone minerals. For example, it is a given that children who are breast-fed in the United

States are smarter than those who are fed infant formulas. However, we also need to ask, how much of that is due to the type of family in which breast-feeding is done? How much is due to the bonding between mother and infant during breast-feeding and how much is actually due to some component (e.g., omega-3 fatty acids such as those found in fish oil) in the breast milk? These types of *confounders* or covariates can be very difficult to sort out when interpreting the medical literature. However, doing so can make the relationships between variables that were otherwise hidden become apparent. The science surrounding bone health involves many confounders which can make it nearly impossible to identify the real causes and effects associated with bone health (Isaacs et al. 2010; Lucas, Chen, and Abrams 1998).

References

A note about references throughout the book: we have provided annotated references. Sometimes these include minimal commentary; and sometimes, more information is included to help the reader decide if it is worth obtaining this reference. When a reference is used in multiple chapters, the annotation will only be provided with the first chapter in which it is used.

This book is intended for a general audience, including both health-care and non-health-care personnel. As such, the referencing is not intended to be as exhaustive as it would be in a scientific paper, but to provide access to the key relevant references. In addition, whenever possible, we have used references that were available online. We feel the relative benefit of identifying such references is more important than always choosing the most well-known reference that readers might have difficulty accessing. Please recognize that some journals, most notably several key nutrition journals, make their articles available for free online free after a fixed time period, usually 1 year after publication. Other articles may be made available free of charge via the National Institutes of Health (NIH) repository after a period of time, as well. Most reference sections in books and articles are not intended for anyone to read them. We have tried to change that paradigm here.

Isaacs EB, Fischl BR, Quinn BT, Chong WK, Gadian DG, and Lucas A. 2010. Impact of breast milk on intelligence quotient, brain size, and white matter development. *Pediatr Res* 67:357–62. Research into brain development and feeding methods during infancy are controversial and challenging areas. However, this study used MRIs to evaluate brain growth based on feeding and suggests that breast milk may be related to brain growth. This type of evidence is not final or completely convincing, but in the future it may help resolve the issue of how to evaluate the effects of feeding approaches, including breast-feeding, on long-term outcomes. (Free online.)

Lavin SR, Chen Z, and Abrams SA. 2010. Effect of tannic acid on iron absorption in straw-colored fruit bats (*Eidolon helvum*). *Zoo Biol* 29:335–43. In zoos, fruit bats get too much iron in their diet and this can cause serious health problems. Adjusting their diet to increase the amount of inhibitors of iron absorption is one possible solution. This study did not harm any of the bats involved. (Not free online.)

Lucas A, Morley R, and Cole TJ. 1998. Randomised trial of early diet in preterm babies and later intelligence quotient. *BMJ* 317:1481–7. This is a very well known study in which it was shown that premature infants receiving breast milk achieved better developmental outcomes than those receiving infant formula. The strength of this study was that infants whose mothers did not provide their own milk were essentially randomized to whether they got human milk. This is very rarely done due to ethical concerns with limiting access to human milk. The study limitations are that the infants were premature and, therefore, the comparisons were made against preterm infants who were fed routine infant formula, rather than infants who were fed the higher nutrient-containing preterm formulas we use now. (Nonetheless, this is a landmark study that is worth reading and is available free online.)

Laing CJ, Trube A, Shea GM, and Fraser DR. 2001. The requirement for natural sunlight to prevent vitamin D deficiency in iguanian lizards. *J Zoo Wildl Med* 32:342–8, www.reptileuvinfo.com/docs/d3-iguanian-lizard-laingand-fraser.pdf. According to the authors, this is, "a thorough understanding of the physiology of vitamin D in other vertebrate groups [that] will help to highlight specific adaptations and assist in our understanding of their implications." Enough said. Go learn about it, and think about it next time you are at the zoo and you see some iguanas hiding out in the shade—or if your child has a pet iguana that does not get enough outdoor time. Actually, vitamin D prevents rickets in rats as well. That is how it was originally tested for efficacy in the 1920s. We are not too worried about rickets in rats. (Free online.)

chapter one

Why does bone health in children matter, and what are the key players in bone health?

We begin by asking these simple questions, "Why does bone health in children matter, and what are the key players in bone health?" After all, everyone knows that children drink a lot of soda (*pop* to those raised in the Midwest and *Coke* to those raised in Texas), and they may occasionally break a bone due to clumsiness or to making heroic efforts to climb where it is unsafe. In the daily battle of raising children, preventing a disease that usually appears 30 or more years after childhood hardly seems a high priority. Furthermore, it is common knowledge that milk is needed for bone health, so other than filling up the fridge with milk that often is not fully consumed, why worry about this issue? Would it not be easier to give children a daily calcium and vitamin D pill and not worry about bone health at all?

Why does bone health in children matter?

We answer this with three separate lines of arguments related to bone and a fourth unrelated directly to bone. The three arguments we will discuss related to bone are:

1. Preventing adult diseases such as osteoporosis, obesity, and hypertension is clearly and undeniably a task that starts in childhood and potentially prenatally. To ignore this is to give a child an unneeded bad start on adult health. We spend a lot of time picking the right schools for our children based largely on their goals for adulthood; it hardly seems unreasonable to do the same for their diet. The idea that osteoporosis begins in childhood has been well recognized in the literature and is a fundamental aspect of our thinking about pediatric bone health (Heaney et al. 2000).
2. Although consequences of bone loss *during* childhood are uncommon, they can occur. Nutritional rickets has made a comeback in the United States in recent years, and although most childhood fractures are not related primarily to nutrition, some are, and can potentially

be prevented (Weisberg, Scanlon, and Cogswell 2004). Rickets is not a benign condition. Its consequences for growth and development are considerable, and although it is a treatable condition, it is much better to prevent it than to treat nutritional deficiencies leading to rickets. It is not an equally distributed burden either. Rickets is more common in African-American infants compared to Caucasian infants (Kreiter et al. 2000). There is no reason for any child, excluding a few with rare congenital problems involving calcium and vitamin D metabolism, to develop rickets. This is a solvable problem and should be solved through education, diet, and nutritional supplementation. Established guidelines for nutritional evaluation and interventions should be developed and implemented. This type of program should be part of a global strategy of health education and clinical care for children.

3. A large number of children and adolescents live with chronic illnesses or are survivors of serious illnesses in childhood. This list includes diseases such as inflammatory bowel disease, cystic fibrosis, and childhood cancer. It also includes eating disorders such as anorexia nervosa that often have severe consequences for bones. Children are often the recipients of medicines, such as steroids, which affect bone directly or are associated with other health issues, including cerebral palsy, congenital disorders, and many others where loss of bone or loss of bone function are serious and common problems (Abrams and O'Brien 2004). Dietary guidelines mostly relate to healthy children, but providing a bone healthy diet is an important challenge for all children.

The fourth argument not related directly to bone is discussed below:

4. There is a real, but still not fully understood possibility that calcium and vitamin D have substantial nonbone health benefits both for children and adults (Holick 2010). There is plausible, but inconclusive, evidence that these nutrients, separately or together, may (1) decrease the risk of excessive weight gain, (2) decrease the risk or severity of some cancers, including colon cancer, (3) decrease the effects or severity of pulmonary diseases, such as asthma, and (4) decrease overall mortality in adults. Identifying and quantifying these nonbone related benefits effects remains challenging. The many advocates for vitamin D's crucial role in achieving these benefits are far from having enough evidence to conclusively demonstrate an effect for many of these outcomes, especially in children. However, for parents and caregivers guiding children now, this developing body of evidence needs to be considered. While the risks are small, the benefits of obtaining even the minimum recommended levels of

calcium and vitamin D may be considerable in areas beyond bone health. That does not mean, however, that high-nutrient intakes are justified without adequate scientific evidence of their safety or efficacy.

Establishing healthy diets begins early. It includes identifying obstacles to obtaining healthful foods such as lactose intolerance and developing healthy dietary patterns that last a lifetime. This includes choosing low-fat dairy products over high-calorie, nutrient-void sodas or dubiously valuable *energy drinks*. Given the already existing database suggestive of multiple beneficial effects obtained from a good calcium and vitamin D status, it is more than reasonable to work towards incorporating these nutrients into the diets of our children in reasonable quantities now, as we await more confirmatory evidence.

Key players in bone health

There is considerable confusion about what are the key aspects of bone health and, particularly, how they relate to each other. Although we will spend a good bit of time going over these throughout the book, let us begin with a brief listing of them and a bit about their physiology as related to bone health.

Calcium

The popular conception is that calcium equals bone. That is, if you have enough calcium, then you have strong bones; and if you have bone problems, it is due to inadequate calcium. The reality is much more complex. For example, one of the most severe congenital diseases of bones is called *osteogenesis imperfecta*. In individuals with this condition, the bones have a reasonably normal amount of calcium; it is the protein matrix that forms the bones that is abnormal. Giving more calcium or vitamin D to children with this condition will not fix it, although therapy to decrease the rate at which calcium is reabsorbed from bones appears to be helpful.

When there is insufficient calcium getting to bones in children, it causes rickets in certain circumstances. This usually happens when calcium intake is extremely low, such as occurs in some countries, especially in Africa. Calcium gets to bones by being absorbed in the intestines and then it is transferred to the bones. This absorption can occur either as mediated (aided) by vitamin D, a process called *active absorption* which occurs through the cells (transcellularly), or via a process that does not require vitamin D, called *passive absorption* in which the calcium moves between intestinal cells (paracellularly). When dietary calcium is high, more absorption is passive, nonvitamin D dependent. When dietary calcium is low or average, more absorption is active, vitamin D dependent.

Vitamin D

It is fully understood that vitamin D is needed for calcium to be absorbed, but vitamin D plays other roles in bone health as well. Vitamin D is transferred to the liver where it is converted into a form called *25–hydroxyvitamin D*, also called *calcidiol*, and abbreviated as 25(OH)D. Then, this form is transferred to the kidney where it is converted to the active form. The active form, 1,25 dihydroxyvitamin D, is called *calcitriol*, and abbreviated as $1,25(OH)_2D$. It is involved in regulating how the intestine, bones, and kidneys handle calcium, as well as other minerals. Note that while calcitriol is the active form of vitamin D, the level of it in the blood is not a good measure of vitamin D status. That is, people who have somewhat low levels of vitamin D in their body can have normal or even high calcitriol levels. The form of vitamin D that is generally most useful for measuring by blood tests is the serum 25(OH)D.

We will spend a lot of time talking about vitamin D and its role in bone health in later chapters. Remember, however, that vitamin D is not a part of bone itself; it is a mediator related to bone mineral metabolism. Vitamin D is not really a vitamin because of its ability to be synthesized with the help of ultraviolet light in the body. It functions in the body more closely as a hormone that allows for many important activities to occur related to bone health and other cellular processes.

Phosphorus

Phosphorus has a mixed image as a bone nutrient. On one hand, phosphorus is bound to calcium and is a fundamental component of the mineral part of bone that makes bones strong. Without enough phosphorus in the diet and the bones, they will be weak and rickets may develop. There is even a rare form of genetic illness that leads to loss of phosphorus from the kidneys and this helps cause rickets. On the other hand, too much phosphorus in the diet, which may result from excess soda consumption, can potentially cause some loss of phosphorus from the bones and weaken them. Phosphorus often gets a bad reputation though it is not usually responsible for harming bone.

Protein

Protein? Why is protein on this list? Protein is really what bone is made up of and minerals like calcium and phosphorus fill up the protein matrix. There is a lot of confusion about whether some types of protein or too much protein is bad for bones. For the most part, and especially for children, this is not really a concern. Good healthy diets with adequate protein are critical to bone health.

References

Abrams SA and O'Brien KO. 2004. Calcium and bone mineral metabolism in children with chronic illnesses. *Ann Rev Nutr* 24:13–32. This is a review of many of the relationships between calcium deficiency and chronic illnesses in children. Not all illnesses are covered, but many of the concepts and discussions of the multiple aspects of chronic illness and bone health are considered. We discuss chronic illness and bone health further in Chapter 8. (Not free online.)

Heaney RP, Abrams SA, Dawson-Hughes B, Looker A, Marcus R, Matkovic V, and Weaver C. 2000. Peak bone mass. *Osteoporos Int* 11:985–1009. Although a bit dated, this detailed review considers the evidence that osteoporosis is a pediatric disease and that building up bone mass during childhood and adolescence is a key aspect of prevention. There is little doubt that we have a genetically programmed peak bone mass, and that we need to do our best to have our children reach it. It is not clear whether maximizing calcium intake is the best way to do that, but going too low, such as well below the Estimated Average Requirement (EAR) is not a good idea. (Not free online.)

Holick MF. 2010. *The vitamin D Solution: A 3-Step Strategy to Cure Our Most Common Health Problem* [Hardcover]. New York: Hudson Street Press. Read it. Do not believe every word of it though. Decide for yourself if he is right or if more evidence is needed before believing that vitamin D is the *solution*. We are unconvinced by many of the arguments in this book, but there is value in being educated about all sides of an issue. Our focus is on pediatrics. Those readers who wish a more detailed understanding of the limitations to the arguments in this book, which is related to adult medicine, will need to look at the Institute of Medicine's (IOM) 2011 report. (Not free online.)

Kreiter SR, Schwartz RP, Kirkman HN Jr, Charlton PA, Calikoglu AS, and Davenport ML. 2000. Nutritional rickets in African-American breast-fed infants. *J Pediatr*.137:153–7. The problem of rickets is due to both low-calcium intake and low vitamin D. These factors are particularly common among African-American infants thereby placing them at the greatest risk. Extended breast-feeding without vitamin D supplementation is often seen in this population. Breast-feeding is great, and we need to encourage it among African-Americans, but the importance of vitamin D supplementation needs to be emphasized in this high-risk group. (Not free online.)

Weisberg P, Scanlon KS, Li R, and Cogswell ME. 2004. Nutritional rickets among children in the United States: Review of cases reported between 1986 and 2003. *Am J Clin Nutr* 80:1697S–705S. We do not really know the incidence of vitamin D or calcium deficient rickets in the United States. There are more reports appearing of children with rickets, but uncertainty exists as to how much this represents better reporting and how much it represents an actual increase. Rickets is not a legally mandated *reportable condition* in the United States, so the Centers for Disease Control (CDC) does not have data on the exact number of cases, what the cause was, and so forth. Furthermore, some cases of rickets are due to diet and some are due to identified genetic problems—so separating these different types when determining the frequency of rickets is nearly impossible. Overall, it would be helpful if state or national surveys tracked the incidence of rickets and the causes. The ongoing National Children's Study (www.nationalchildrensstudy.gov/) may be helpful in this regard. (Free online.)

chapter two

How do we identify and quantify dietary requirements?

We begin by asking some basic questions about dietary requirements. What is a Dietary Reference Intake (DRI) and what is a Recommended Dietary Allowance (RDA)? How do we assess the needs for calcium, phosphorus, other minerals, and vitamin D? The heart of this discussion involves developing an understanding of the new guidelines for calcium and vitamin D that were released on November 30, 2010, and published in 2011 by the Institute of Medicine (IOM 2011).

The language of dietary requirements

To understand dietary requirements, we must first understand *the language* of dietary requirements. This language is not intuitive and even those trained in dietetics and nutrition are often uncertain of the meaning of the nutritional guideline terms. Physicians receive essentially no training in this area and often do not understand the implications of the different terms as they are related to healthy individuals versus those with acute and chronic illnesses.

The terms used in dietary intake recommendations for vitamins and minerals in the United States and Canada are shown in Table 2.1 with the most recent values for calcium and vitamin D provided by the Institute of Medicine (IOM 2011) shown in Table 2.2. DRI values are an umbrella term for all dietary requirements based on age and gender. The Estimated Average Requirement (EAR) is the value of a nutrient such that 50% of the population will have sufficient intake to meet their nutritional needs. RDA is the value of a nutrient needed for almost all (97% to 98%) of the population to meet their nutritional needs. This is the number that generally should be used when an individual's diet is evaluated for adequacy. If there is not enough scientific evidence to determine an RDA, then an Adequate Intake (AI) is used. Finally, the Upper Limit (UL), or, more formally, the Tolerable Upper Intake Level, is the maximum amount that will not pose health risks for almost all healthy people. These values make up the alphabet soup of acronyms and terms used by the nutrition community to assess nutrient recommendations. A comparison of key guidelines from the previous (1997) DRI values to the 2011 values is shown in Tables 2.3 and 2.4.

Table 2.1 Dietary Reference Intake (DRI): Daily Nutrient Recommendations Based on Age and Gender; Set at Levels to Decrease the Risk of Chronic Disease

Estimated Average Requirement	EAR	Value to meet the needs in 50% of individuals. At this level, the remaining 50% would not meet their nutritional needs. The EAR is used to set the RDA.
Recommended Dietary Allowance	RDA	Recommended daily levels of nutrients to meet the needs of almost all (97% to 98%) healthy individuals in a specific age and gender group; used when there is scientific consensus for a firm nutrient recommendation.
Adequate Intake	AI	Similar to RDAs, and used for nutrients that lack sufficient scientific evidence to determine a RDA.
Tolerable Upper Intake Level	UL	Maximum intake that most likely will not pose risks for health problems for almost all healthy people in that age and gender group.

Guideline development: The Institute of Medicine (IOM)

Whereas it is nice to have simple statements of dietary requirements, the nutrition community has recognized for some time that more complex guidelines are needed. The Food and Nutrition Board (FNB) of the IOM has developed guidelines for nutritional intake by individuals in the United States and Canada for many decades. The IOM (http://www.iom.edu) "is an independent, nonprofit organization that works outside of government to provide unbiased and authoritative advice to decision-makers and the public." That the IOM is not a government organization, but an independent group that receives support from government agencies, is often not understood. The reports issued by the IOM inform public policy, but are not "laws" or even Food and Drug Administration (FDA) rules. They are informative guidelines that are used by many organizations, including federal agencies and Congress, in developing public policy.

In 1997, the IOM established guidelines for calcium and vitamin D intakes in the United States and Canada (IOM 1997). These guidelines also included magnesium, fluoride, and phosphorus because these nutrients are also critical for bone health and it was thought that packaging these nutrients together when developing these guidelines was a reasonable thing to do. The guidelines, however, especially those for vitamin D, were felt to be out-of-date by many, and a careful review of the evidence

Table 2.2 Dietary Reference Intakes (DRIs) for Calcium and vitamin D

Life Stage Group	Calcium			vitamin D		
	EAR (mg/day)	RDA (mg/day)	UL (mg/day)	EAR (IU/day)	RDA (IU/day)	UL (IU/day)
Infants 0–6 months		200*	1000		400*	1000
Infants 6–12 months		260*	1500		400*	1500
1–3 years old	500	700	2500	400	600	2500
4–8 years old	800	1000	2500	400	600	3000
9–13 years old	1100	1300	3000	400	600	4000
14–18 years old	1100	1300	3000	400	600	4000
19–30 years old	800	1000	2500	400	600	4000
31–50 years old	800	1000	2500	400	600	4000
51–70 year old males	800	1000	2000	400	600	4000
51–70 year old females	1000	1200	2000	400	600	4000
>70 years old	1000	1200	2000	400	800	4000
14–18 years old, pregnant/ lactating	1100	1300	3000	400	600	4000
19–50 years old, pregnant/ lactating	800	1000	2500	400	600	4000

Source: Institute of Medicine, Dietary Reference Intakes for Calcium and Vitamin D, Washington, DC: National Academies Press, 2011.

* For infants 0–12 months of age, the Adequate Intake (AI) is used rather than the EAR or RDA.

suggested that it was time to revise the recommendations (Yetley et al. 2009). The decision to reevaluate the 1997 vitamin D recommendations was neither made quickly nor without careful consideration of the rationale for such a review.

It might be thought that it is rapid and relatively inexpensive to create an IOM review. In reality, the type of review done by the IOM often takes up to two years to conduct and may cost several million dollars. It is simply not possible to do such a review frequently or without good reason. Furthermore, attempting to change the RDA annually or every couple of years for all nutrients would lead to chaos. Numerous programs use the RDA and other DRI values in order to determine dietary content. This includes many government programs such as the Special Supplemental Nutrition Program for Women, Infants, and Children, commonly referred

Table 2.3 Calcium Dietary Reference Intakes (DRIs) by Life Stage (Old versus New)

Life Stage Group	1997[a] AI (IU)	2011[b] EAR (IU)	2011[b] RDA (IU)
0–6 months	210	200 (AI)	—
7–12 months	270	260 (AI)	—
1–3 years old	500	500	700
4–8 years old	800	800	1000
9–13 years old	1300	1100	1300
14–18 years old	1300	1100	1300
19–30 years old	1000	800	1000
31–50 years old	1000	800	1000
51–70 year old males	1200	800	1000
51–70 year old females	1200	1000	1200
71+ years old	1200	1000	1200
≤ 18 years old, pregnant	1300	1100	1300
19–50 years old, pregnant	1000	800	1000
≤ 18 years old, lactating	1300	1100	1300
19–50 years old, lactating	1000	800	1000

Note: Values shown are the recommended daily calcium intakes by life stage group. EAR is the Estimated Average Requirement and RDA is Recommended Dietary Allowance.

[a] Institute of Medicine, Food and Nutrition Board: Dietary Reference Intakes for Calcium, Phosphorus, Magnesium, Vitamin D, and Fluoride, Washington, DC: National Academy Press, 1997.
[b] Data from Institute of Medicine. Dietary Reference Intakes for Calcium and Vitamin D, Washington, DC: National Academies Press, 2011.

to as the WIC program. It is not practical or appropriate to change these values either frequently or without very good indication that there is scientific evidence that was not available when the previous guidelines were developed. Note that a decision to reevaluate DRI values does not mean they *will* be changed. It only means that new science exists that is believed to be important and novel such that the current DRI values should be carefully reevaluated. It would be nice if all of the DRI values were reevaluated regularly, such as every 5 years. However, financial constraints make this an unrealistic goal.

The IOM process

The IOM forms its panels for making recommendations through a process in which potential committee members are nominated, or self-nominated, and they are then reviewed by senior members of the IOM who select the final committee. In general, IOM panels consist of experts that cover

Table 2.4 Vitamin D Dietary Reference Intakes (DRIs) by Life Stage (Old versus New)

Life Stage Group	1997[a] AI (IU)	2011[b] EAR (IU)	2011[b] RDA (IU)
0–6 months	200	400 (AI)	—
7–12 months	200	400 (AI)	—
1–3 years old	200	400	600
4–8 years old	200	400	600
9–13 years old	200	400	600
14–18 years old	200	400	600
19–30 years old	200	400	600
31–50 years old	200	400	600
51–70 year old males	400	400	600
51–70 year old females	400	400	600
71+ years old	600	400	800
≤ 18 years old, pregnant	200	400	600
19–50 years old, pregnant	200	400	600
≤ 18 years old, lactating	200	400	600
19–50 years old, lactating	200	400	600

Note: Values shown are the recommended daily vitamin D intakes by life stage group. EAR is the Estimated Average Requirement and RDA is Recommended Dietary Allowance.

[a] Institute of Medicine, Food and Nutrition Board: Dietary Reference Intakes for Calcium, Phosphorus, Magnesium, Vitamin D, and Fluoride, Washington, DC: National Academy Press, 1997.

[b] Data from Institute of Medicine. Dietary Reference Intakes for Calcium and Vitamin D, Washington, DC: National Academies Press, 2011.

a broad range of areas within the topic of interest. Members are usually selected who have not made strong public statements about the likely outcome of the panel. This issue is often confusing for many people. They wonder why the 2011 Calcium and vitamin D Panel for example, did not include several well-known vitamin D experts.

We do not know the answer with respect to specific individuals, and it is inappropriate for us to speculate on individual panel member choices. The decision-making process related to the suitability of individuals to serve on such a committee is properly not a matter of public record. There are far more possible applicants for an IOM committee than available positions.

The IOM Panel on Calcium and vitamin D operated as a consensus panel. That is, the final conclusions had to be agreed upon by every member of the committee. This means that members had to be able to compromise in reaching final verdicts even if they did not all necessarily believe that each number in the final DRI value was the perfect choice. IOM panels must include individuals with knowledge of the nutrients being studied for a wide range of ages, as well as experts in nutritional policy and epidemiology. Therefore, not all members would necessarily have focused expertise on vitamin D physiology in adults, for example.

The IOM members for the Calcium and vitamin D Panel were not paid with the exception that they received public acclaim that came from their work. (See for example: http://www.vitamindcouncil.org/news-archive/2010/vitamin-d-council-statement-on-fnb-vitamin-d-report/.) Well, not exactly *overwhelming* acclaim. Often, IOM panel members are senior scientists or actively practicing physicians who donate a large amount of their time working on the IOM report. This is time during which they are not seeing patients or conducting their usual research. It is an honor to be named to one of these committees, but it requires a lot of time and the support of one's hospital or medical school to provide the time needed to serve on an IOM panel.

IOM panel members must discuss any conflicts of interest they have in the original selection process and during the initial panel meeting. It is not necessary that panel members have no financial relationship with any group having an interest in the topic of the panel. That would be almost impossible to do for many topics because experts have often done research supported by companies or nonprofit groups related to their field of expertise. Rather, panel members must disclose these conflicts and have the IOM leadership evaluate them. They must also discuss conflicts of interest with the other committee members.

Once an IOM dietary guideline panel is formed, it holds a series of meetings to develop the new guidelines. Usually, at least one of these meetings is a public forum in which both invited scientists and the public are allowed to comment on the issues at hand. The public meeting related to the 2011 Calcium and vitamin D Panel was held on August 4, 2009. Although not widely known, virtually every presentation from that meeting has a handout available free of charge to the public. (Visit: http://www.iom.edu/Activities/Nutrition/DRIVitDCalcium/2009-AUG-04.aspx and enjoy the range of opinions under the heading entitled "Presentations.") In addition to this public meeting, panels hold a number of private meetings to discuss the research and develop a conclusion. These discussions are not available for public review.

As noted, the IOM process is neither fast nor inexpensive and this was true for the current 2011 Calcium and vitamin D Panel. Fourteen scientists met in Washington, DC eight times, reviewed the literature, and wrote the report which was then extensively reviewed. This was a process that took almost 2 years. One advantage to this careful and detailed approach is that it provides much information that can be used by many people to understand the physiology involved. A big disadvantage is that it is impossible to make *quick* changes to a DRI value even during the time period that the panel was meeting.

Let us suppose there is a new compelling research study that some-one (often the study's author) believes should change the DRI values, and this study is released a year after the panel concludes its work. There is no mechanism for the IOM to review the study rapidly or without forming another committee. The original committee is deactivated immediately upon the release of their report. They cannot just look at a new study and change their mind, or revise the dietary guidelines that were released in their name. Furthermore, this is probably not a good idea to do anyway. One study coming out today suggesting certain changes may be reversed by another study the following week. Quick changes in dietary guidelines are not good public policy.

After the IOM makes its determination of the new DRI values, they are then sent with the text of the rationale for the values to a fairly large number of reviewers. Reviewers are chosen from across the spectrum of people with opinions about the issues at hand. These reviewers may include those who hold strong opinions about what the DRI values should be. Then, the reviewers send their written comments back to the IOM. These comments are confidential, and reviewers have been told that their comments will be kept confidential. The identity of the reviewers are not known to the committee members until the time of the final release of the DRI guidelines, and at no point are particular comments linked to indi-vidual reviewers by name.

When the IOM receives the reviews, every single comment made by a reviewer is evaluated. An independent team, including a scientist not involved in the panel or the review, evaluates these comments. Major criti-cisms of the IOM draft report require a response from the IOM commit-tee. These responses are sent to an IOM review team that determines if they are acceptable. A key issue that is not well understood, especially with respect to the 2011 DRI Panel for Calcium and vitamin D, is that the IOM committee is not required to *convince* the original reviewers of the correctness of their opinion and how they responded to the review-ers' comments. The reviewers' opinions must receive a response from the committee acceptable to the IOM review team, but it is not a back and forth process between the reviewers and the IOM committee.

This is often a problem because reviewers or other people could expect the IOM process to be conducted the same way a journal article is reviewed. A scientific or medical journal article is almost always reviewed by at least one, usually two or three peer-reviewers. These comments and criticisms are sent back to the journal editor who usually forwards them to the original authors. The authors must respond, and typically, for important comments, there is communication back and forth between the reviewer and the author, until both sides are, at least, reasonably satisfied. At times, there is never satisfaction. That is, the reviewer never thinks the author's response is acceptable, and in such cases, the editor must make a final decision regarding who is correct and whether the manuscript should be published.

In the IOM process for the DRI guidelines, the reviewers do not have a chance to see and respond to what the IOM committee said in response to their criticisms. The IOM process does not include such an interchange. As such, there can be some confusion and misunderstanding about what the review contained, and why individuals who were ultimately identified publically as reviewers did not have their views and criticisms reflected in the final document.

The DRI guidelines provide a range of intake recommendations and also thoroughly review the medical literature and issues related to the nutrients being evaluated. These guidelines are needed to answer the questions listed above and to provide guidance not just to individuals, but also to provide recommendations for population intakes to those who are planning institutional food packages or creating public policy related to food. The IOM released its new guidelines for calcium and vitamin D on November 30, 2010. However, as the official publication date of these guidelines is 2011, they are referred to as the 2011 IOM Guidelines for Calcium and vitamin D (IOM 2011). The actual guidelines are contained in a several hundred page book that is available free of charge online, but requires page-by-page downloading. You may find key summaries, reviews (Ross 2011a; Ross 2011b; Abrams 2011) and harsh criticism of the guidelines (Heaney and Holick 2011) to be more helpful and take less time to review. The new guidelines may be found in the Table 2.1 through Table 2.4.

Other approaches to dietary guidelines

Different groups use very different approaches to providing dietary recommendations. For example, the American Academy of Pediatrics (AAP) stated in a 2009 position paper that "all infants and children require 400 International Units per day (400 IU per day) of vitamin D beginning soon after birth" (Wagner 2008). This statement sounds clear and easy to understand and provides direct guidance for practicing pediatricians. But, it leaves out a lot of important information. For example, does it apply to all children, whether they are healthy or not, premature or full-term? Does it apply to children beginning the day after birth or does "soon" mean a couple of weeks or even months? Most importantly, does it really mean exactly *400 IU per day*, or would 350 IU per day be close enough? Would 500 IU per day be too much? Do you have to get the 400 IU every day or would it be okay to get 380 IU one day and 420 IU the next day? What about 2800 IU every week? What form of vitamin D is needed? Should it only be vitamin D_3 or is vitamin D_2 okay?

How can we compare these dietary guideline terms to recommendations such as those of the American Academy of Pediatrics (AAP)?

In general, those (e.g., physicians, registered dietitians, nurse practitioners and physician assistants) who provide advice about nutrient intakes will advise individuals to have an intake at about the RDA for the nutrient. This intake level will assure that nearly all individuals meet their biological needs without any significant risk of toxicity. We will discuss the specific values used for children for calcium and vitamin D throughout this book. The types of guidelines issued by the AAP and other organizations are generally intended to be similar to the RDA. That is, they are intended as an intake that is safe and effective for nearly all individuals. However, whereas the RDA guidelines have specific definitions and mathematical derivation, this may not be the case for more general nutritional intake recommendations.

It is important not to overread such recommendations. A calcium intake of 1300 mg per day, whether a DRI value, or a statement by the AAP, has a substantial variability attached to it. Both are general target values, not exact requirements. When these values are misinterpreted, the most common flaw is that there is an exact cutpoint of nutrient intake which defines deficiency.

If an adolescent consumes 1290 mg per day of calcium and the guidelines say they should get 1300 mg per day, is this a real problem?

An important issue in interpreting dietary guidelines and population intakes is the idea of achieving an exact intake stated in the recommendation. When someone says that teenagers need 1300 mg per day of calcium, it is easy to look at population data and decide how many of them are not meeting this exact value. This approach has been widely used, for example, to indicate a crisis in calcium intake among teenage girls because about 90% do not have an intake of 1300 mg per day of calcium.

However, this type of analysis is vastly oversimplified and not as meaningful as it sounds. First of all, the data generated to come up with the 1300 mg recommendation is not very precise. It could be that teenagers do fine on 1200 mg or that some need 1400 mg daily to meet their needs. It has recently been suggested that up to 1600 mg of calcium are needed daily by this age group (Heaney 2011), but this analysis is not consistent with the approach to dietary calcium recommendations used by the IOM. Furthermore, there is no difference between a daily calcium intake of 1290 mg and one of 1310 mg. Such exact cut points of intake to define deficiency are not very accurate or helpful. Not only is there no meaningful difference physiologically between the two intakes, but there is no way to determine a person's dietary intake of any nutrient that accurately on a daily basis without sending a registered dietitian to observe them. However, even the presence of a dietitian would cause a bias because the person would know they were being observed and likely change what they were eating since nobody likes to eat a Snickers bar right in front of a dietitian!

Even if we could measure the number of servings someone consumed exactly (by weighing all of their food), then using the food label still is not a very accurate way of determining actual intake of vitamins and minerals. The food label generally represents the minimum amount of the micronutrients actually in the food. Many, if not most foods, contain more than the labeled amount in order to ensure that the micronutrients do not go below the amount listed on the food label during the time the food is on the shelf before it is eaten. In other words, if the label says a food has 200 mg of calcium, it could easily have 220 mg, and it may have even more than that. This can be a problem for vitamin D especially, and independent testing labs have confirmed that both foods and supplements are often far off the mark from their labeled amounts. Other methods of determining intake such as using computer software programs based on the U.S. Department of Agriculture (USDA) nutrient database are more accurate and less time-consuming than using food labels for this purpose.

The problem of determining actual intakes confounds almost all nutrition research, especially in children, and makes for dietary recommendations that are imprecise. When home-cooked meals are taken into consideration because many children eat them, this can be a particular problem. The reality of determining what people actually eat is subject to many errors. When dealing with children, these errors can be readily magnified.

Nutritional status markers

When it comes to figuring out bone mineral and vitamin D related issues in children, we have to look at what are called *status markers*. Status markers are the biological outcomes that can be measured and used to tell us whether someone has enough of a nutrient in their diet. Sometimes, these are relatively easy to determine, sometimes not.

Status markers can be specific to one nutrient; for example, the serum (blood after the red cells and plasma are removed) level of phosphorus, or they can be integrated measurements reflecting the nutritional status of multiple nutrients, as would be the case for a Dual-Energy X-ray Absorptiometry (DXA) scan of bone mineral content or density. Status markers can be closely related to diet, such as the serum phosphorus or have a very limited relationship with diet, such as the serum calcium. They also may not even be an actual dietary substance, such as vitamin D, but a blood value of something made in the body that uses the vitamin or is derived from it such as the serum 25(OH)D. Other examples of this in nutrition would include hemoglobin, hematocrit, and serum ferritin as related to iron intake. When dealing with minerals, it is often the case that the serum value is a poor marker of overall mineral status. Magnesium and zinc are two key minerals whose serum values indicate an idea of status, but the markers are especially limited in identifying mild nutrient deficiency.

Vitamin D levels

Before considering more specifics of nutrient requirements, it is important to discuss the vitamin D value, what it is, and what are the areas of knowledge and lack of knowledge about it.

Vitamin D is either absorbed via the diet or converted in the skin from previtamin D via ultraviolet B (UVB) radiation from the sun. It is then transported to the liver where it is converted to 25hydroxyvitamin D, 25(OH)D. This form of the vitamin is then transported to the kidney where it is converted to 1,25 dihydroxyvitamin D. Research on each of these forms is extensive and ongoing. Much of the physiology is described in detail in the IOM report (IOM 2011; Ross et al. 2011b) in addition to many texts and is not covered here. Our purpose is to discuss the clinical importance of these forms of vitamin D as they relate to the health of children.

Classically, serum 25(OH)D is the primary circulating form of vitamin D that reflects the overall amount of vitamin D in the body. Some new research challenges this idea and suggests that other forms of vitamin D are also important, including the native compound. Nonetheless, considerable evidence for every age group shows that the serum 25(OH)D fairly accurately reflects the exposure someone has to vitamin D. That is, it distinguishes between people who have had little vitamin D exposure (via sunshine or diet) and those who have had more. This relationship may be more complex in the case of obesity where vitamin D and its metabolites that are stored in fat cells are not identified by the serum 25(OH)D testing. The half-life of serum 25(OH)D in the blood is generally thought to be about 3 weeks (Shils and Shike 2005), although some evidence suggests that it may be shorter in patients with inflammatory conditions such as inflammatory bowel disease.

Much less certain, however, is how good a marker serum 25(OH)D is of *functional* outcomes related to vitamin D. That is to say, is someone who has a high serum 25(OH)D going to have health benefits that someone with a low serum 25(OH)D will not have? The standard answer that is given is "yes" and, therefore, many people are advised to have their serum 25(OH)D measured and to target specific values of serum 25(OH)D to ensure a healthy outcome (Holick 2011). However, the accuracy of this answer is far from clear despite the strong advocacy for it.

Table. Selected percentile values for serum 25-hydroxyvitamin D (25OHD), by sex and age, and by pregnancy and lactation status in females: United States, 2001–2006

Characteristic	n	5th	10th	25th	50th	75th	90th	95th
				Serum 25OHD (nm ol/L) percentile				
				Male				
Age (years)								
1–3	581	40.7	48.3	58.2	69.5	84.4	94.7	101.0
4–8	970	42.6	47.8	58.0	67.3	78.8	92.0	99.9
9–13	1,473	32.5	40.4	49.9	62.1	74.5	87.4	98.5
14–18	1,978	25.3	33.0	45.7	58.5	71.2	84.9	95.7
19–30	1,611	23.0	29.4	41.9	55.3	68.7	83.6	94.3
31–50	2,244	25.1	31.3	44.2	57.4	71.5	84.5	94.3
51–70	1,853	25.6	32.7	44.1	58.1	71.3	83.7	91.8
Over 70	1,217	25.4	31.7	44.6	57.2	69.7	82.7	90.1
				Female				
Age (years)								
1–3	584	43.3	49.8	58.5	68.3	79.4	89.2	94.9
4–8	989	38.4	44.2	54.5	67.2	80.0	93.4	101.0
9–13	1,515	27.7	34.6	46.3	57.6	68.4	80.9	87.5
14–18	1,823	20.8	27.2	41.1	57.2	71.6	87.1	104.0
19–30	1,346	18.5	25.4	40.0	55.9	76.2	95.6	111.0
31–50	2,097	19.2	25.3	38.9	55.3	71.0	87.6	101.0
51–70	1,866	21.2	27.0	39.7	54.7	69.7	85.4	93.4
Over 70	1,197	22.6	27.1	40.5	55.5	69.6	84.1	93.6
Pregnant or lactating	1,067	24.5	31.4	44.5	62.4	78.2	94.7	109.0

Source: CDC/NCHS, National Health and Nutrition Examination Survey (NHANES), 2001–2006; data for ages 1–5 years from NHANES 2003–2006.

Figure 2.1 Serum 25(OH)D status of persons aged 1 year and over: U.S. 2001–2006. This figure is from the CDC report showing the values of 25(OH)D in Americans. It is useful as it shows the distribution of values clearly. To understand this tabular form of the results, look for example at the value for males age 1–3 years. There were 581 children in this age range who were tested. The median value (not the average) was 69.5 nmo/L. This can be divided by 2.5 to get the more usual units of ng/mL—in this case, 27.8 ng/mL. Note that 5% of children in this age group have a value below 40.7 nmol/L which is 16.3 ng/mL. (Data from Looker AC, Johnson CL, Lacher DA, Pfeiffer CM, Schleicher RL, and Sempos CT, 2011, Vitamin D Status: United States, 2001–2006, *NCHS Data Brief* March (59):1–8. Free online.)

This is especially true in children for whom it is difficult to identify health benefits of specific levels of serum 25(OH)D. We consider this issue in detail in Chapter 5. It is important to look in an unbiased way at the science behind determining what serum 25(OH)D levels are needed for healthy children. Data collected from a national survey called the National Health and Nutrition Examination Survey (NHANES) found that most Americans over 1 year of age have sufficient serum 25(OH)D levels based on the IOM guidelines (Figure 2.1).

Interpreting serum 25(OH)D levels

It is certainly true that many studies have been reported over the past several years linking low levels of vitamin D, as reflected by the serum 25(OH)D, to an increased incidence of different diseases. However, it is not true that a cause and effect have clearly been demonstrated for most of these conditions. Several populations have lower serum 25(OH)D levels but that does not mean this is due to a disease. For example, almost any child with a chronic illness is likely to spend less time outside in the sun and have a lower level of serum 25(OH)D. Individuals of ethnic and racial groups with darker skin absorb less UVB and have lower vitamin D levels because of it. However, this does not mean that higher rates of some diseases seen in these populations are caused by low vitamin D status.

This situation, in which the endpoint (a disease or condition) points to the presumed cause such as vitamin D deficiency, is called *reverse causality* and it may be important in understanding the possible link between measured vitamin D levels and many diseases or other conditions (Welsh, Peters, and Sattar 2011).

The only way to be sure about cause and effect, and especially to know if we should be giving children a lot of vitamin D, is to conduct controlled trials that include enough participants to answer the questions being asked. These trials need to be conducted in virtually every case before we draw firm conclusions about the value of a specific nutritional intervention for either healthy or sick individuals. When considering children, the study must either be specifically done in children of the appropriate ages, or at least include some children in the overall study population where appropriate. It has been commonly claimed that such research is impossible or not worth doing. We do not agree. As will be discussed in Chapter 13, these studies are difficult and often expensive to conduct. However, it is exactly this type of research that often shows us how our preconceived notions are not correct. The classic example of this is vitamin E, in which controlled trials did not confirm many of the benefits to health attributed to it from earlier studies. Controversy remains regarding numerous nutrients for this reason.

The Food Label

There is a tremendous amount of debate right now about how to provide consumers with meaningful and accurate information about the nutritional quality of foods they choose. This is a topic for a book in itself, but we would like to discuss a few issues specific to bone health.

The Nutrition Facts *Food Label* is that area in the shape of a box found on most foods sold in the United States and

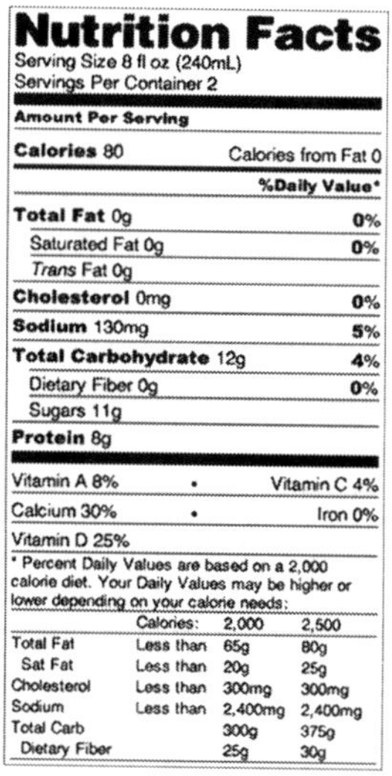

Figure 2.2 An example of a typical food label in the United States.

throughout the world (Figure 2.2). It contains information about the nutrient content of foods. The content of the food label is very tightly regulated by the FDA based on long-standing rules and policies that are extremely difficult to change in a practical way. Even the smallest changes in rules, for example, mean that every company has to redo all of its packaging, and this can take many years to do and cost millions of dollars. So, changing food label rules is not done on a whim and is a massive endeavor.

Having said that, food labels in the United States are woefully inadequate. This is especially true for vitamins and minerals. The food label only tells you the percentage each serving of food has of something called the *Percent Daily Value* (%DV). By FDA rule, the food label does not, and *cannot* actually tell you how much (i.e., mg content) of the vitamins or minerals, such as calcium and vitamin D, it actually contains. Supplement pill labels can tell you this on their label; food labels cannot. In fact, the IOM formed a panel to look at this and similar issues. In 2003, the panel concluded, among other things, that the "absolute amounts should be included in the Nutrition Facts and Supplement Facts boxes for all nutrients" (http://books. nap.edu/openbook.php?record_id=10872&page=5). We are still waiting (Institute of Medicine 2003). It is hard to understand why this has not been implemented more than 8 years after the recommendation was made by the IOM. Several other countries include the absolute amounts, some in multiple languages (http://www.foodcentsprogram.com.au/about-foodcents/ shop-smart/labels/). Until the food label is changed, Americans will need to learn how to use them as best they can to choose healthy and nutritious foods, mostly by using the Daily Value.

So, what is the Daily Value and where did they get the values? Well, for most nutrients they chose the highest RDA values for any age group over the age of 4 years from the 1968 RDAs. This is correct, the 1968 values. It is as if we have learned nothing about nutritional requirements in more than 40 years! Forget anything we have learned in more than 4 decades about nutrition; it is not reflected on the food label as it currently exists in the United States. Of course, the same IOM panel that recommended including the amount of nutrients, recommended numerous fixes for this issue as well (IOM and FNB 2003). We are not holding our breaths waiting for these changes to be implemented either.

What is worse is that the 1968 RDA values are not even used as the Daily Value in some cases, such as calcium. For calcium, the 1968 RDA was 1200 mg. It was decided that was not a good number so they chose 1000 mg for the Daily Value to make a nice even number. Yes—the Daily Value for calcium is basically a made-up number.

The bottom line is that the Daily Value, and the percentage of it that is contained in any food, is only useful if (a) the population knows what the values are, (b) it is understood that the Daily Values are designed for comparison shopping, not detailed dietary planning, and (c) people understand the Daily Values in terms of how many servings of food they are going to consume. Since the public understands virtually none of this, then the Daily Value concept is highly flawed. Food labels need to be revised to include the actual amount of the mineral or vitamin that is contained in each serving.

However, despite all of these flaws, the Daily Value has another use. It is the basis for the claim that a food is a *Good Source* or an *Excellent Source* of the nutrient. This concept is also highly flawed and poorly understood. For example, if you buy a steak, it is a great source of iron. Not only that, but the iron is heme iron and highly bioavailable which means that it is readily absorbed and available for hemoglobin incorporation. The consumer has no way of knowing this however since steaks (and fresh fruits and vegetables) do not have food labels or even percent Daily Values.

On the other hand, high-sugar containing cereals can add a small amount of vitamin D and make these claims on their packaging. To be a Good Source, you need to have 10% of the

Daily Value, and to be an Excellent Source, 20%. Cereal with a ton of sugar and high in calories can claim to be a Good Source of vitamin D by providing exactly 40 IU of vitamin D in a serving. However, more than 40 IU of vitamin D is often provided by the milk, which is consumed with the cereal!

Interpreting the Medical and Nutritional Literature on Calcium Supplementation

When reading the medical literature, and especially the lay press, it is important to understand the substantial limitations associated with what is presented there. Those who conduct and publish scientific studies have a very strong bias towards finding and publishing positive medication or interventions related to significant effects of what they are researching. Negative findings are frequently hard to publish and even harder to garner media attention. Furthermore, when results are published, even from controlled trials, there is a tendency to focus on the positive outcomes and ignore the negatives.

Here is an example to show what we mean. Let's forget about vitamin D for a minute and discuss calcium in teenagers. There have been numerous trials focused on giving teenagers calcium supplements to see if the supplements improved their bone mineralization. Many of these have been well-conducted controlled trials in which the supplement was compared to a placebo. But, there are lots of flaws in these studies that limit their interpretation.

The biggest flaw is something called the bone-remodeling transient (Heaney 2001). In this process, adding more calcium into bone causes the rate at which calcium leaves bone, called bone *resorption,* to slow down. The net effect is an increase in bone mineralization. This affects children and adults, and makes almost every relatively short-term calcium supplementation study look like a winning answer.

The problem is that this effect is mostly temporary. The bones start adapting to the higher calcium intake, and the supplement has a much smaller or nonexistent long-term effect. In rapidly growing bones, there may be some benefit, but for many ages, including most adults, calcium supplementation has relatively little effect when looked at over several years, instead of 6 months—the typical time span for a research study.

In a 7-year supplement study, a group of investigators looked to see if giving calcium to preteen girls would improve their bone mineralization (Matkovic et al. 2005). Before the study, the investigators predicted what benefit they might expect to find and determined how many girls had to be in each group. After 7 years they looked at the data and found that what they had decided would be a meaningful increase in bone mineralization in advance of the study had not, in fact, occurred. However, they did find a tiny benefit that was statistically significant for a few outcomes. So, this is what they focused on when they published in a major nutrition journal. The media press release touted these positive findings and ignored the fact that the study was basically a negative. That is, the study had not shown what it set out to show and the limited positive findings might well represent changes that are not physiologically important. What media would want to hear that? Or hear that after 7 years, there was virtually no benefit to an intervention like giving children a calcium supplement?

Most studies on calcium supplementation have either failed to look for long-term benefit, or looked and found a minimal one, if any. In adults, we are beginning to suspect that high-dose calcium supplementation has more risk of cardiovascular harm than any bone health benefit. This does not mean that a good calcium intake, especially from diet, is not important. It does mean that we should be very dubious about claims for benefits for high-dose (e.g., more than 500 to 1000 mg per day) calcium supplement pills for most people.

This issue is very common and can be seen in many *reviews* of topics. If there are 100 studies published about something, and half are positive and half are negative, then reviewers with a bias will find a reason to ignore the ones they do not like. Combine that with the tendency to publish only the positive studies, and there is a chance for a huge bias unless a true *systematic* review is done, and even that has its limitations.

One of the oddities, in our view of nutrition, is the tendency to believe in nutritional solutions without requiring the type of evidence that is expected of pharmaceuticals. One hears consistently about foods or nutrients that will prevent or cure diseases. The FDA and Federal Trade Commission (FTC) have only limited power to combat such excesses and even when they can, the power of the Internet is such that the claims go unregulated.

For example, consider *coral calcium*. A quick Internet search brought up a mere 6 to 37 million hits for this term depending on the search engine used. It takes seconds to find a claim like "coral calcium—an ionic source of calcium that provides the body with upwards of 95% to 100% absorption!" (accessed August 2011, http://www.calcium-factor.com/). A recent search of a health food supplement store found a whole shelf filled with so-called *coral calcium*.

Now, this is complete nonsense. There is absolutely no form of calcium that has been shown to be 95% absorbed in a human being. The use of biologically important sounding words like *ionic* and *absorption* does not change the fact that calcium, even highly soluble sources, are generally absorbed at about 30% to 40% to a maximum of 60% to 80% in populations with extremely low calcium intakes (Vargas Zapata et al. 2004). Yet, people spend a lot of money to buy these sources without any evidence of benefit compared to standard calcium. The FTC took action against some of these marketers (http://www.ftc.gov/opa/2004/01/barefoot.shtm), but the ads still remain easily accessible.

Finally, one has to recognize that advocacy for high-dose nutritional supplementation, and accusations that someone is trying to hide the benefits are easy to make, easy to spread, and are often made by people with a compelling ability to make these points. Who does not want to believe that there is a conspiracy of doctors to not prevent horrible diseases like cancer and that a simple vitamin pill can prevent cancer? Interestingly, doctors themselves often get caught up in this. When studies come out that do not support their viewpoint or even suggest the opposite, few are interested in hearing it. Furthermore, the *negative* side is rarely as effective or as willing to use the media to make a negative case against a miracle nutrient.

So, as we begin to look at different ages of children and bone health, we will try our hardest to be fair brokers and look at both sides. In many ways, this is much easier to do with children than adults, as the evidence and research are more limited, and thus, controversies are often easier to evaluate. Still, few have looked at this topic critically and perhaps fewer want to read a book that does not have a miracle cure as its theme.

Ultimately, however, we are guided by a *first do no harm* approach. This applies to both pharmaceuticals and nutritional supplements. As such, we believe that scientifically based, unbiased research is critical. Especially, in dealing with the nutritional needs of children.

References

Abrams SA. 2011. Dietary guidelines for calcium and vitamin D: A new era. *Pediatrics* 127:566–8. This is a short summary of the key issues specific to pediatrics based on the IOM 2011 Report. (Not free online.)

Heaney RP. 2001. The bone remodeling transient: Interpreting interventions involving bone-related nutrients. *Nutr Rev* 59:327–34. The overwhelming majority of calcium supplementation studies are highly flawed as they are too short-term. Any intervention helps bones in the short-term, what are needed are long-term studies. This review explains why.

Heaney RP. 2011. The nutrient problem, as seen through the lens of calcium. *J Clin Endocrinol Metab* 96:2035–7. This is an editorial supporting the idea that up to 1600 mg of calcium is needed daily by adolescents. Editorials are a great way to deliver opinions that, although peer-reviewed, often are not as carefully scrutinized as typical peer-reviewed articles. In this case, there are numerous statements about the dietary guidelines and IOM process, and a perspective about individuals needing very high-calcium intake that we do not agree with. However, opinions are interesting, editorials get widely quoted, and these are often what we take away from the literature as it is easier to quote an editorial than to read the details of the article on which it was based.

Holick MF, Binkley NC, Bischoff-Ferrari HA, Gordon CM, Hanley DA, Heaney RP, Murad MH, and Weaver CM. 2011. Evaluation, treatment, and prevention of vitamin D deficiency: An endocrine society clinical practice guideline. *J Clin Endocrinol Metab* 96:191130. The Endocrine Society has its views in favor of widespread serum 25(OH)D screening for nearly half of the U.S. population. The authors suggest testing about half of all Americans for their vitamin D level. Who will pay? What is the evidence that this screening, by far the largest such screening program ever proposed for a single nutrient, would have any health benefits for children or be worth the billions spent on it compared to providing low-cost health insurance for the same children? Why would you pick Hispanics as a group for targeted screening? This group encompasses many people from multiple backgrounds, many of whom do not have dark skin and are not shown to be widely at risk for vitamin D deficiency. More discussion of this reference is found in Chapter 5. (Not free online.)

Heaney RP and Holick MF. 2011. Why the IOM recommendations for vitamin D are deficient. *J Bone Miner Res* 26:455–57. Tell us how you really feel, guys. Do not hold back. Among a number of reasons these authors have for thinking the IOM did not get it right is the view that ancient humans had very high levels of vitamin D via sunshine exposure, so we should too. Whether this is meaningful or not is debatable. It is not clear what specific benefits ancient humans got from their high level of sunshine exposure and they are not available to ask. This does not strike us as a compelling argument since our lifestyle and diet is not much like those of our ancient ancestors.

Institute of Medicine and Food and Nutrition Board (FNB). 2003. *Dietary Reference Intakes: Guiding Principles for Nutrition Labeling and Fortification*. Washington DC: National Academy Press. This book contains some very interesting and at times controversial information about nutrition labeling and food fortification guidelines from the Institute of Medicine. Note that most of these recommendations have not yet been turned into action by the U.S. or Canadian governments. (It can be downloaded page-by-page for free online.)

Institute of Medicine. 2011. *Dietary Reference Intakes for Calcium and vitamin D.* Washington, DC: National Academy Press. This is the long version. It is much easier to get the key points by reading the Ross et al. paper in *J Clin Endo Metab* (see below). However, for those who wish to really understand the committee and how it derived the new DRI values, it is worth purchasing and reading the entire text. (You can download it page-by-page free online or at least the summary pages.)

Institute of Medicine and Food and Nutrition Board. 1997. *Dietary Reference Intakes for Calcium, Phosphorus, Magnesium, vitamin D, and Fluoride.* Washington, DC: National Academy Press. In 1997, the IOM put out guidelines for calcium and vitamin D. The 1997 report is mostly useful in a historical context now, although the guidelines for magnesium, phosphorus and fluoride remain the current ones and have not been revised since the 1997 report. (Available free of charge online via the Institute of Medicine Web site.)

Matkovic V, Goel PK, Badenhop-Stevens NE, Landoll JD, Li B, Ilich JZ, Skugor M, Nagode LA, Mobley SL, Ha EJ, Hangartner TN, and Clairmont A. 2005. Calcium supplementation and bone mineral density in females from childhood to young adulthood: A randomized controlled trial. *Am J Clin Nutr* 81:175–88. A massive controlled trial of calcium supplementation in girls during adolescence. Actual results showed no real effect, although the conclusion of the paper made it appear there was one. Ultimately, this is an inconclusive study and even less helpful in current thinking about bone health because vitamin D was not a part of the evaluation. It is unlikely that a study like this will ever be repeated, and if it is repeated, there would need to be careful control of everything from vitamin D intake and status to other nutrients important for bone health and exercise.

Ross AC, Manson JE, Abrams SA, Aloia JF, Brannon PM, Clinton SK, Durazo-Arvizu RA, Gallagher JC, Gallo RL, Jones G, Kovacs CS, Mayne ST, Rosen CJ, and Shapses SA. 2011a. The 2011 dietary reference intakes for calcium and vitamin D: What dietetics practitioners need to know. *J Am Diet Assoc* 111:524–7. This is an explanation of the DRI values written for dietitians. (Not free online.)

Ross AC, Manson JE, Abrams SA, Aloia JF, Brannon PM, Clinton SK, Durazo-Arvizu RA, Gallagher JC, Gallo RL, Jones G, Kovacs CS, Mayne ST, Rosen CJ, and Shapses SA. 2011b. The 2011 report on dietary reference intakes for calcium and vitamin D from the Institute of Medicine: What clinicians need to know. *J Clin Endocrinol Metab* 96:53–58. (Free online. This is a great price and has all of the key information in one article.)

Shils ME, Shike M et al. 2005. *Modern Nutrition in Health and Disease*, 10th ed. Philadelphia, PA: Lippincott Williams & Wilkins. This book covers it all, not just vitamin D. (Not free online.)

Vargas Zapata CL, Donangelo CM, Woodhouse LH, Abrams SA, Spencer M, and King JC. 2004. Calcium homeostasis during pregnancy and lactation in Brazilian women with low calcium intakes: A longitudinal study. *Am J Clin Nutr* 80:417–422. What happens when women have extremely low calcium intakes during pregnancy? The body learns to absorb virtually all of the calcium and ultimately both mom and baby do okay from a bone perspective. This is not ideal and may be even more problematic with a high-salt U.S. diet. Nonetheless, the capacity for adaptation by increasing calcium absorption is remarkable.

Wagner CL, Greer FR, and American Academy of Pediatrics, Section on Breastfeeding and Committee on Nutrition. 2008. Prevention of rickets and vitamin D deficiency in infants, children, and adolescents. *Pediatrics* 122:1142–52. [Published correction appears in 2009. *Pediatrics* 123:197.] This is the AAP view of vitamin D requirements. It is slightly different than the IOM. However, the differences are not large. The statement in this document that serum 25(OH)D levels should exceed 32 ng/mL in pregnant women is inconsistent with the 2011 IOM Report and much of the available data. (Free online.)

Welsh P, Peters M, and Sattar N. 2011. Vitamin D in rheumatoid arthritis: A magic bullet or a mirage? The need to improve the evidence base prior to calls for supplementation. *Arthritis Rheum* 63:1763–9. More information is needed before vitamin D is a magical cure according to these authors. We agree. There is no such thing as a magic bullet. (Not free online.)

Yetley EA, Brulé D, Cheney MC, Davis CD, Esslinger KA, Fischer PW, Friedl KE, Greene-Finestone LS, Guenther PM, Klurfeld DM, L'Abbe MR, McMurry KY, Starke-Reed PE, and Trumbo PR. 2009. Dietary reference intakes for vitamin D: Justification for a review of the 1997 values. *Am J Clin Nutr* 89:719–27. The decision to have the IOM look again at vitamin D requirements was not random, but a carefully considered and expensive decision. This manuscript provides a very useful insight into the decision-making process about dietary requirements. (Free online.)

chapter three

Infants

As we begin our march through childhood and discuss developmental changes in bone growth and mineralization, it is worthwhile to start with a brief history. After all, it was the condition of rickets seen in infants and young children that began the search for a preventative agent, vitamin D, and the quest to make children have strong bones for life.

Rickets: A historical perspective

Rickets was first identified in the 1600s. Although some of the early history is vague, it was initially thought to be, in part, a breathing problem because children with the condition would be weak with poor rib cage support. This led to coughing, pneumonia, and, sometimes, to fatal respiratory failure. Rickets was associated with the urbanization of society and more indoor time during the industrial revolution in Europe. It was not until the 1920s that investigators identified vitamin D and ultimately isolated it in the 1930s as an agent that could prevent and treat the condition. Although historical data are not clear, it is stated that up to half of children in both the United States and parts of Europe had rickets during some historical eras, including the late 1800s. Similar claims are made for parts of Europe after World War I. Milk was irradiated to provide vitamin D beginning in the early 1930s, which had a tremendous effect on decreasing the incidence of rickets (Figure 3.1).

An interesting historical aspect is that the addition of vitamin D to milk and similar products did not occur right after its discovery. Vitamin D was even patented at one time, although ultimately that patent was not held as viable since it had been recognized that vitamin D synthesis could occur from sunshine exposure. One early product that was fortified with vitamin D was beer. In 1936, Schlitz beer with the *sunshine vitamin* was marketed providing 400 IU of vitamin D per can of beer (Figure 3.2). Sadly, they dropped that product fairly quickly, but one wonders if it could come back, although this would not help us much in pediatrics.

Currently, even carbonated soda products can be vitamin fortified, and it would not be inconceivable for the government to allow just about any food or beverage to have vitamin D added to it. Whether this is a good idea or not is debatable. One concern with any unregulated program of adding vitamins or minerals to food sources is the possibility

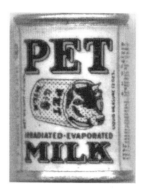

Figure 3.1 Evaporated milk can from the 1930s, showing irradiation to provide vitamin D.

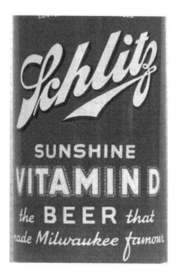

Figure 3.2 What a great idea! Add vitamin D to beer. Probably would not help children much, but sounds like a creative idea. Unfortunately, this product was dropped from the marketplace in the late 1930s.

of excessive intake if too many foods are fortified, or if the fortification levels are excessive. Another concern is that adding vitamins to unhealthy foods does not make them healthy, and there can be confusion about this amongst the public, especially children.

Rickets: Clinical features and X-ray findings

First, it is important to understand a little bit about rickets. Rickets is a condition in which bones are inadequately mineralized. It occurs when there are not enough of the bone minerals, especially calcium and phosphorus, being deposited into the bones as they are growing. The bones must still be growing for rickets to occur (Craviari et al. 2008; Ozkan 2010). There is no such thing as adult-onset rickets; the closest adult-onset equivalent is a condition called *osteomalacia*, and it is not exactly the same.

Rickets usually occurs in infants and toddlers, especially children who are about 6 months to 2 years of age. It can occur in older children, and even in young adolescents. However, it is uncommon in the first 3 months of life. This is primarily because the mineralization of bones *in utero* is not regulated by vitamin D, and is fairly constant, unless there is severe failure of the feto–placental unit.

Clinically, rickets is recognized by the presence of a number of common physical signs, including bowing of the legs and abnormalities of the skull (Figures 3.3 and 3.4). It is diagnosed by X-ray findings that are specific to the condition, but do not identify the cause. Very suggestive biochemical tests exist, such as the serum alkaline phosphatase activity, but the final diagnosis relies on the X-ray findings, which are similar regardless of the age of the child (Figures 3.5 and 3.6).

In looking at these X-rays, radiologists focus on the ends of the bones. They look for abnormalities in which the bones do not have discrete edges, but have what looks like frayed endpoints. These are called *cupping* and *fraying* of the metaphyses, and they are characteristic of rickets. Other common X-ray findings include a widened area between bones. In particular, note that one can see both on X-rays and by directly looking at a severely affected child, a bowing of the long bones. Fortunately, this usually heals with therapy, and currently surgery is not usually needed. However, rickets may delay or prevent walking and may have life-long consequences for mobility if not properly identified and treated.

Although it is generally thought that rickets is due to not enough vitamin D, this is an oversimplification. Rickets occurs when inadequate calcium and phosphorus are available for growing bones to mineralize. As such, it can be caused by any health problem that limits these minerals from reaching the skeleton while it is growing. Vitamin D is converted in the kidneys from 25(OH)D to its biologically active form of 1,25(OH)$_2$D, which allows for dietary calcium to be more readily absorbed. However, calcium can be absorbed without vitamin D. If there is enough calcium in the diet, then some, but not all of the effects of vitamin D deficiency on calcium absorption can be overcome. Similarly, even with the highest levels of vitamin D, if there is a severe shortage of calcium, then rickets can occur. This type of rickets is due primarily to calcium, not vitamin D deficiency, and is common in parts of Africa, as well as in premature infants.

Let us look at rickets and bone health in infants. We will first discuss premature infants, then healthy breast-fed full-term infants, and lastly older infants in the second six months of life.

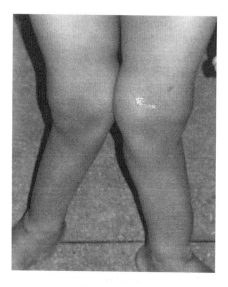

***Figure* 3.3** Photo of a small child in Jos, Nigeria with rickets and bowed legs. (Photo courtesy of Thomas Thacher, M.D.)

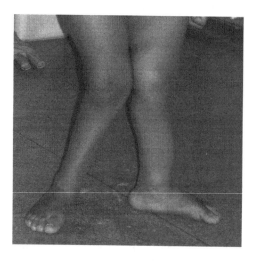

***Figure* 3.4** Additional photo of a small child in Jos, Nigeria with rickets and bowed legs. (Photo courtesy of Thomas Thacher, M.D.)

Premature infants

Premature infants are a special case since the bones of premature infants grow very quickly compared to full-term infants. Premature infants are often fed in a different way than full-term infants because they need specialized feeding approaches due to their small size and immature

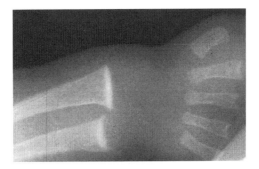

Figure 3.5 X-ray of a premature infant with clinical rickets. Ends of bones have characteristic bucket shape (cupped) and are nondistinct.

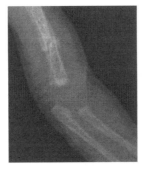

Figure 3.6 X-ray of a premature infant with clinical rickets and a fracture. The etiology of these fractures is very often uncertain and may be related to routine handling in small infants with undermineralized bones.

intestines. However, since more than 12% of all infants are born prematurely (before 37 weeks gestational age) in the United States, and about 1% are born very low birth weight (VLBW) at < 1500 g, or about 3 pounds 5 ounces, this is not a rare problem. This also gives us a chance to talk a bit about mineralization of bone *in utero*, or before birth.

   In utero, the fetus is mostly water, with almost all of the bone being formed in the third trimester. At birth, the full-term newborn has about 30 grams (30,000 mg) of calcium in its skeleton (Abrams 2007). Of this, about two-thirds was transferred across the placenta from the mother during the last trimester of pregnancy. The rate it enters the skeleton reaches a peak of about 110 to 120 mg per kilogram (kg) per day at about 32 to 36 weeks gestation. Since the 32- to 36-week fetus weighs about 1.8 to 2.5 kg, then a total of about 200 to 300 mg of calcium must come across the placenta into the skeleton of the fetus every day.

Neonatologists are tremendously concerned about adequate bone health, especially in preterm infants because they are vulnerable to fractures due to their size. Fractures are often noticed incidentally on X-rays taken for other purposes, or by an unexpected swelling of an arm or a leg. The causes of these fractures are multifactorial; it is not just because the baby is small. In preterm infants, bones are growing faster than they are mineralizing leading to a risk of undermineralization and fractures. Additionally, the care that often needs to be provided in a neonatal intensive care unit (ICU) can lead to an accidental fracture. A broken bone in a 2-pound baby can occur very inadvertently while moving the baby and can be caused by a doctor, nurse, or family member.

After the birth of a VLBW infant, one goal of neonatal management is to try to come as close as possible to providing the infant with the same amount of minerals they would have received if they were still *in utero*. This is particularly important as the preterm infant grows from about 1000 grams (2 pounds 3 ounces) to about 2000 grams (4 pounds 5 ounces). Breast milk from mothers who deliver prematurely is somewhat special and, at least, initially has many benefits for the preterm infant. For example, it has extra protein to help growth, and lots of biologically active factors to help develop the intestine, increase feeding tolerance, and protect from severe bowel diseases that can occur in premature infants. Unfortunately, human milk, even from a mother who delivers her baby prematurely, does not have extra amounts of calcium in it. This is not changed if the mother is supplemented with high amounts of calcium and vitamin D.

Since breast milk usually has about 30 mg of calcium in every 100 milliliters (mL) of milk (or 0.3 mg per 1 mL), and premature babies typically take in about 150 mL per kg of body weight, then the most calcium that the preterm baby can take in from breast milk is about 45 mg per kg body weight each day (150 x 0.3). Calcium in breast milk is well absorbed, but a typical baby absorbs at the most about 60%. In other words, about 60% of the 45 mg per kg that is ingested is absorbed. The body must also urinate some calcium, usually about 3 to 5 mg per kg per day in preterm infants. So, when calculating this, we find the net amount of calcium available for bone growth in an exclusively human–milk–fed preterm infant is at most about 22 to 25 mg per kg per day. This is less than one-quarter of the requirements of a premature baby for bone growth, and it puts them at risk for rickets due to inadequate calcium for the skeleton (Mitchell et al. 2010).

It also appears, but this has not been shown for certain, that most of the calcium that is absorbed by the preterm infant in the first weeks of life is absorbed via the nonvitamin D dependent *passive* route (Bronner et al. 1992). Even if the possibility existed of the intestine absorbing 100% of the calcium in human milk, then the total amount absorbed would be nowhere near the amount needed to meet the bone growth needs of very premature infants. This cannot be changed even with high-dose vitamin D supplementation. Vitamin D helps to absorb calcium, but it cannot make the body absorb more than 100% of the dietary calcium, or even close to 100% of the calcium in the diet.

Therefore, despite the enthusiasm of some for high doses of vitamin D in preterm infants, the fundamental problem with achieving adequate bone mineralization in premature infants is one of providing enough calcium and phosphorus. Some people recommend up to 1000 IU per day of vitamin D for premature infants (Rigo et al. 2007), although the evidence for a benefit to vitamin D intakes above 200 to 400 IU per day is probably minimal when these infants are fed formulas or fortifiers used in the United States.

In neonatal nurseries, special products called *human milk fortifiers* (and special types of infant formulas) are used to increase the amount of both calcium and phosphorus needed for bone mineralization by the infant. These products also include supplements of other important components for bone health, including magnesium, zinc, and protein. The use of these products has led to a marked decrease in rickets in preterm infants compared to before their introduction over 30 years ago. However, infants who have major health problems cannot always tolerate these fortified feedings or infant formulas, and rickets remains a fairly common neonatal ICU problem. As the preterm infant gets bigger, there may be some benefit to adding some extra vitamin D to the usual amount in their fortifiers and formulas, but there is no question that rickets is almost exclusively a mineral (calcium and phosphorus) problem in most preterm infants.

In developing countries, access to human milk fortifiers is more limited as they can be expensive and not readily obtained. In some cases, infant formulas designed for preterm infants can be used as fortifiers for addition to human milk. However, the problem of rickets in preterm infants is more common in resource-poor international settings, and it remains an area in which we are actively interested in conducting research to determine the best way to provide needed minerals to these infants.

Feeding premature babies after they go home

A baby is considered *preterm* if delivered before 37 completed weeks gestation, or, in simple terms, if born more than 21 days before its due date. But that covers a lot of territory. The majority of babies born at 25 weeks (or about 3 months earlier than their due date) will survive, and some born at 22 to 23 weeks, and especially many born at 24 weeks, will survive. There is a large difference in how babies who are born at 24 weeks grow after they come home than one born at 36 weeks, yet both were considered premature or preterm.

The failure to distinguish this difference in many recommendations leads to a lot of confusion, both for parents and for health-care providers. Also, whereas most infants at 36 weeks can be breast-fed completely from birth and do not spend extra time in the hospital, this is certainly not true of infants born at less than 34 to 35 weeks.

Let us consider small infants, especially those born at less than about 4 pounds (1800 g). These babies often go home with bones that are still not fully mineralized to the level seen in babies born full-term. If breast-fed, it is commonly recommended to either fortify some feeds with powdered formula or to provide one or more feedings each day as a high-calorie, high-mineral formula. This is especially true for babies born at less than 1500 g birth weight (about 3 pounds 5 ounces).

An important question in babies this small is, "How long do we need to continue to use specialized formula or supplement mother's breast milk?" The general answer is that this should continue until the baby is clearly growing on the growth curve once it is corrected for prematurity. When possible, a goal of reaching about the 25th percentile for weight, length, and head circumference should be sought before stopping specialized feeding practices at home. In *bigger* babies in this group, this may only be for about 2 to 3 months after going home or the original due date. For the smallest babies, it may be for 8 to 9 months after the original due date. There is no *one size fits all answer*. The good news is that, at least from a bone perspective, infants will catch-up fairly quickly to where they should be based on their size, with the catch-up generally occurring by 1 to 2 years of age.

Bigger preterm babies are a different story. When we consider babies born over about 4 pounds, or at 34 to 36 weeks gestation (often called *late preterm* infants), then at the time they go home, they are likely to have fewer nutritional deficiencies that have built up during their hospitalization. Most of the time, infants who are born at more than 4 pounds and more than 34 to 35 weeks gestation can just be breast-fed at home without concern for their bone health. It is important to watch these babies a bit more carefully than full-term infants to make sure they do not become severely jaundiced or have trouble getting enough milk in the first week of life. Sometimes, they have more trouble learning to breast-feed and it can be helpful to have a lactation consultant involved to help if there are any problems.

In the case of formula-fed babies, then, generally, routine formulas made for full-term infants are adequate for bigger preterm infants; although in some cases, a pediatrician or neonatologist may choose to use a formula designed for home-feeding of preterm infants for the first 2 to 3 months at home. From a bone health perspective, there should be no problem with any reasonable feeding approach, including the use of only breast milk or only routine formula. The use of specialized formulas such as soy formulas or lactose-free formulas for premature infants should be avoided, even if the infant seems to have some spitting or colic symptoms. These formulas have little if any value for preterm infants, and the minerals in them may not be absorbed as well as from those formulas intended for full-term infants or the specialized formulas used for preterm infants after hospital discharge.

Full-term infants

Rickets is very uncommon in the first 3 to 4 months of life in full-term infants. Calcium is deposited into the skeleton of the fetus independent of vitamin D status, and even babies born with very low vitamin D levels do not usually have rickets. Rickets tends to develop beginning at about 3 to 4 months of age. The most common time for clinical rickets is towards the end of the first year of life and early in the second year of life.

The amount of calcium in breast milk is fixed at about 200 mg each day, and this is constant even in mothers with low dietary calcium intake and in mothers who are making enough milk for twins. Typically, a baby consumes about 800 mL (about 27 ounces) of breast milk each day by the second month of life. For twins, lactating women increase their production to twice that. The milk for twins has about the same nutritional content as the milk for one baby. This is how wet-nursing was possible in the past as well. Of historical note, however, is the possibility that the calcium in milk decreases somewhat in the second 6 months of nursing, although the change is not large. A mother who is wet-nursing a second infant might provide slightly less calcium to the second baby than the first baby. It has been postulated that this might have been in part responsible for early rickets in the 17th century, which was believed to be more common among babies being wet-nursed (Thacher et al. 2007; Swinburne 2006). Somewhat surprisingly, taking calcium supplements does not have much of an effect on the amount of calcium in breast milk. Furthermore, mothers in Africa and other areas of the world with very low amounts of calcium in their diet do not increase their milk calcium with supplements (Jarjou et al. 2006).

Now, we do not really know exactly how much of the 200 mg of calcium that is in mother's milk relies on vitamin D in order to be absorbed, and how much is absorbed passively between the cells without needing vitamin D to do so. What we do know is that since bones are pretty well-formed at birth, regardless of the mother's (and therefore the newborn's) vitamin D status, it usually takes time and growth for a clinically apparent mineral deficiency to occur.

Based on the current data, what appears most important is to make sure that no matter what diet the lactating mother has, the infant gets vitamin D early in life so that by 6 to 8 weeks old, the vitamin D level in the baby is adequate to make sure that adequate absorption occurs.

It may seem strange, but there are essentially no data to determine the exact amount of vitamin D needed by babies, whether this amount goes up during the first year of life, and what serum level of 25(OH)D is needed by infants to make sure they absorb vitamin D. Part of the reason there is so little data on infants is that these issues are extremely hard to research in babies. It is not easy to measure the absorption of minerals, including calcium, in the body, and it is particularly hard to do in infants (see Chapter 13). Methods of doing this that include giving intravenous nonradioactive tracers of minerals or that involve prolonged fecal collections are completely safe for infants, but a challenge to perform accurately. It is not ethically acceptable to withhold vitamin D in a research study: and it is impossible, even in the best of circumstances, to study the same baby multiple times during infancy (with numerous blood draws, fecal and urine collections, and X-rays). No parent would allow that.

So, often we have to settle for using evidence obtained from older children, from a few studies looking at bone mineral density, and from the clinical evidence related to rickets. All of these data are hard to sort out because some studies included only breast-feeding infants, some only formula-fed infants, and some included mixed-fed infants.

What are the recommendations for calcium and vitamin D in healthy full-term infants in the first 6 months of life?

To understand the recommendations of the American Academy of Pediatrics (AAP) regarding vitamin D intake and of the IOM regarding calcium and vitamin D intake in the first 6 months of life, we have to consider the historical evidence and the more recent science (IOM 2011). Historically, a vitamin D daily dose of 400 IU prevented rickets in virtually all infants. This level of vitamin D intake was established as the recommendation in the United States in the 1940s with little change since then.

In 1997, the IOM chose to lower the recommendation to 200 IU each day based on the idea that this amount would be enough to prevent rickets. This was the *Adequate Intake* (AI) for vitamin D. As we have noted, this is more than the amount found in breast milk. It was the amount in about one-half a milliliter of most liquid vitamin drops designed for infants. In response to this, the AAP also changed its recommendation to 200 IU per day, but added the proviso that these oral drops did not need to be started until 6 weeks of age. This time period was set because of the concern about making mothers give anything to their infant other than breast milk and the unlikelihood of rickets in the first six weeks of life.

Since then, the AAP has again changed its position and they went back to 400 IU per day beginning *soon after birth* (Wagner, Greer, and AAP 2009), and the IOM, in its 2011 recommendation, similarly went back to the older recommendation of 400 IU per day beginning early in life. It is a good idea for mothers to learn how to give vitamin D drops and begin them in the first days of life. For the most part, the drops are not critical to the baby's health at that stage, but it is a good point in time for the mother to get used to giving them to breast-fed babies.

The recommended 400 IU per day is probably a slightly high estimate of what is needed for most infants, especially those whose mothers are not severely vitamin D deficient. An average intake of about 300 IU per day for the infant is almost certainly enough to ensure adequate vitamin D in the first year of life. Therefore, parents do not need to be too worried about missing an occasional day of giving vitamin D supplements.

However, the reason that the recommendations went back to 400 IU per day from both the AAP and the IOM was related, in part, to concerns about some infants being born with extremely low amounts of vitamin D in their body, as evidenced by low serum 25(OH)D. In general, this is not a problem in terms of the baby's bones at birth, but this evidence of undetectably low levels of vitamin D in some infants and their mothers at birth is worrisome. It was determined that the dose of 400 IU per day was a better idea to ensure a more rapid increase in vitamin D levels in all babies. There was no reason to go tinkering with what had worked for almost 100 years.

As far as calcium is concerned, the IOM continued to support using the amount of calcium in breast milk as its guide and the IOM 2011 panel rounded this amount to 200 mg per day. There is no evidence for any problem related to the calcium intake of breast milk during the first 6 months of life in full-term healthy infants.

The second 6 months of life and early signs of rickets

What we call nutritional rickets is primarily due to a deficiency of vitamin D in the body. To understand this, one has to look at how bone is formed in infancy and what role different levels of calcium and vitamin D have in its formation.

Calcium and phosphorus are transferred to the fetus throughout pregnancy and congenital rickets is rare, but it can exist with extreme maternal vitamin D deficiency. Rickets remains uncommon before 6 months of age, except in babies who have been born very preterm or other infants who have had major health problems limiting their ability to tolerate a normal diet. There are also some rare genetic diseases causing rickets that we will not be discussing in this book, but require diagnosis and treatment by experts such as pediatric endocrinologists or geneticists. Nutritional rickets does, however, begin to develop at about 6 months with a peak in the United States between 6 to 18 months of age.

First, here is a bit of information about the epidemiology of rickets. Rickets is not a legally mandated reportable condition in the United States. That means that there is no law requiring a physician or other caregiver to report that they are treating a child with rickets to the government. Therefore, there are no reliable numbers on how many children actually get rickets each year in the United States. Even if there were such a list, it would be hard to sort the causes, such as prematurity, from the types of rickets seen in older children.

Nonetheless, over approximately the last 10 years, there is little doubt that there has been a substantial resurgence of clinical rickets in the United States, and that this has occurred throughout the country. In understanding this phenomenon, it is important to recognize that there is no one factor that is responsible, but a combination of issues that lead to the problem. Rickets occurs because not enough calcium is provided for the growing skeleton, and the bones are growing without being adequately calcified. In order for calcium to go to the bones, it has to be in the diet and be absorbed from the diet. There also cannot be any health issues in the child that prevent the calcium, once absorbed, from going to the bone. We discuss the effects of chronic health problems in children and bone health in Chapter 8.

The second 6 months of life is a time of relatively rapid bone formation. The amount of calcium needed each day by the skeleton is about 80 to 100 mg. Note that this is much less than the amount that is used by the skeleton of the preterm baby (or third trimester *in utero* fetus), which is 200 to 300 mg per day. Overall, as with preterm infants, about 60% of the calcium in breast milk is absorbed by the full-term infant. Typically, a lactating woman produces about 200 mg each day of calcium in her milk. So, about 120 mg are absorbed (200 mg x 60%) and about 20 to 40 mg are excreted daily in the urine and sweat by the baby. This supplies 80 to 100 mg net of calcium to the baby's bones each day, just as we indicated was needed for bone growth. Interestingly, these numbers do not change a whole lot from about 2 months of age until a year or so of age. Thus, to meet the 80 to 100 mg required, the baby needs to have about 200 mg of calcium in their diet so that 200 mg times 50% absorbed results in 100 mg with 20 to 40 mg lost in the urine as shown in Figure 3.7. Sweat loss should be pretty small in infants. Note that the values shown in Figure 3.7 are for calcium. In general, the values for phosphorus are similar, but they are about one-half the amounts in each case as for calcium.

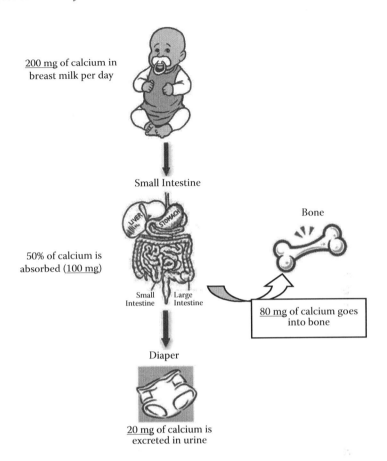

200 mg of calcium in
breast milk per day

Small Intestine

Bone

50% of calcium is
absorbed (100 mg)

Small Large
Intestine Intestine

80 mg of calcium goes
into bone

Diaper

20 mg of calcium is
excreted in urine

Figure 3.7 Flowchart of calcium distribution from diet to bones in an older infant. The typical breast-fed infant consumes about 200 mg of calcium each day from about 800 mL of breast milk. About half of that is absorbed and about half comes out in the stool. Another 20 mg comes out in urine, leaving about 80 mg for the bones. These calculations are not exact and do not take into account sweat loss, but give a general idea of what happens to calcium from the diet as it goes into the body.

No one is really certain what the least amount of calcium is in 24 hours worth of human milk that would be the minimum needed for bone health or would be found in healthy populations of women throughout the world. Calcium excretion into breast milk is tightly regulated. It is likely that a lower value is about 150 mg per day in otherwise healthy mothers, regardless of the mother's calcium intake or her vitamin D status. Now at 150 mg per day, the baby would need to increase absorption to about 70% to get the same amount of absorbed calcium. As previously stated, 70% is nearly the absolute maximum that it is physiologically possible to absorb from any calcium source.

Next, we need to consider factors that might keep the baby from absorbing the 50% to 70% of dietary calcium they need in order to meet that minimum 80 mg per day of calcium going to bone. The most important factor would be the presence of very inadequate amounts of vitamin D. To achieve this high level of calcium absorption during the second six months of life, the infant must have enough circulating vitamin D. This is not so clear during pregnancy. During pregnancy, calcium absorption from the mother's diet also increases markedly, but it appears from both animal and human studies that this is only partly, if at all, related to vitamin D, even though the active form of vitamin D increases in pregnancy (Fudge and Kovacs 2010). This is discussed in more detail in Chapter 7.

So, what are the limiting factors for vitamin D that loom in the 6 to 12 month age period? The most important is not enough dietary vitamin D. Rickets can almost completely be avoided with the use of 400 IU per day of vitamin D. That was known by 1930. In fact, even 200 to 300 IU per day is enough to prevent clinical rickets in most, if not all infants, especially those in the United States. But, breast milk usually only provides about 20 to 60 IU per day of vitamin D. This is biologically a nearly meaningless amount. That means that if the vitamin D drops are not given to an infant, then the only other option is sunshine exposure to form vitamin D in the skin. We will not enter a debate here on the pros and cons of using sunshine as a source of vitamin D: that issue is covered in Chapter 10. However, we can say here that many infants simply do not have much sun-related vitamin D exposure. Infants who have dark skin form less vitamin D in their skin than infants with a light skin color. Combine this with the use of sun block, the effects of wintertime with less outdoor time and less UVB, and add a bit of covering up the skin, a touch of pollution, and we have a *perfect storm* for vitamin D deficiency.

There is no clearly established value of serum 25(OH)D that is so low that calcium absorption does not occur at all. Studies in adults suggest that with a serum 25(OH)D value less than 10 to 12 ng/mL, there is a drop-off of calcium absorption which could lead to a high risk of rickets if maintained for several months. No one really knows how many infants in the United States are below this level; but, based on the available data, it can be reasonably estimated to be about 1% to 3% of non-African-American infants and about 4% to 8% of African-American infants. Multiply this by more than 4 million infants in the United States, about 12% to 14% of whom are African-American (and other groups who have dark skin), and we can come up with a risk pool of up to 100,000 infants. About one-quarter of infants in the United States (about one-eighth of African-Americans) are still primarily breast-fed at 5 to 6 months. This would give us a pool of maybe 20,000 or more at-risk infants. We need one more number here.

That number is the percentage of mothers who are breast-feeding who give vitamin D drops to their baby. That is one of the easiest numbers to find out. It is about 12% (Perrine et al. 2010). Now we have a group of many thousands of babies at serious risk for vitamin D–deficient nutritional rickets in the United States each year.

What an amazing number! A disease completely solved in 1930 might affect many thousands of babies in the United States and be a near miss with potential clinical effects in thousands more. Although we derived this number from theoretical concerns, it fits well with the clinical experience throughout the United States in Childrens' Hospitals and other clinics. We have thousands of cases of a severe, life-altering disease that is completely preventable.

What should be done?

So, we have to consider how to approach this problem. The IOM and the AAP are uniform in their recommendations that *all* infants receive vitamin D supplementation of some form, including drops for breast-fed infants. Yet, as we noted, only about 12% of breast-feeding mothers provide those drops. Why? Surely even the most contentious issues in medicine rarely have only 12% of parents doing what is recommended.

The impediments to getting families to give their infants vitamin D drops are numerous (Table 3.1). First, is the genuine belief of many parents and pediatricians that they are not necessary for a healthy, full-term infant. For decades, the recommendations from many groups, including the AAP were that only *high-risk* infants needed vitamin D. This seemed to work, but in reality, there were always some cases of rickets in infants who needed the drops but did not receive them. What

Table 3.1 Reasons Why Breast-Fed Babies Do Not Get Vitamin D Supplements—Even Though It Is Recommended by the AAP and Many Other Groups Throughout the World

- Many *parents* think breast milk has everything the baby needs and do not accept that their baby may have a need for vitamins.
- Some *pediatricians* do not think it is necessary either. Babies will get what they need from sunlight and breast milk.
- Some think, "Why bother now?" With the exception of a few kids with rickets (who are high-risk anyway), babies are getting the same vitamin D that they have always gotten. "What's the big deal?"
- Some parents think formula is better than breast milk so they do not need extra vitamins.
- Added expense. In most states vitamin D drops are not covered by insurance or federal assistance programs.
- Added hassle. Babies do not like having to take the vitamins.

made the situation *explode* was the marked increase in breast-feeding in the 1980s and 1990s without a simultaneous increase in the frequency of vitamin D supplementation.

There are some mothers and doctors that just do not like the idea of anything other than breast milk being given to an infant. They are concerned that if vitamins or iron are deemed necessary for babies then mothers will not breast-feed or will stop breast-feeding. This concern is not entirely without merit. Recent surveys of several population groups have suggested that a substantial portion of mothers think that infant formula is better for their baby nutritionally than breast milk or that some formula should be given.

The resolution of this concern is actually explaining the need for the vitamin drops to mothers. A simple, "give these drops to your baby" is completely inadequate as an explanation for families. Of course, for this to happen, pediatricians and others who see newborns and small infants must themselves believe in the need for vitamin D drops. We need more aggressive education for everyone in this regard. We must also be clear that giving a breast-fed baby vitamin drops does not mean that breast milk is inadequate or that formula is better.

Perhaps a written handout from pediatricians, family medicine physicians, nurse practitioners, midwives, obstetricians, and others would be effective. A text might say something like this:

> Dear Mother of Breast-Fed Newborn:
>
> Congratulations on your beautiful and healthy new baby and for choosing to breast-feed your baby. Your milk has all of the nutrition needed to make your baby grow and thrive. It is the perfect food for your baby. However, your baby will need vitamin D drops to make sure your baby's bones grow strong. Vitamin D can come from being out in the sun. But we don't recommend you rely on this for your baby. Instead, we strongly advise that you begin these supplements in the next week for your infant and give them daily. Do not use highly concentrated vitamin D drops. Check with your caregiver or pharmacist in selecting a vitamin D or multivitamin drop.

The second problem is that, in most states, vitamin D drops are not available in public assistance programs such as Medicaid or via the WIC program. Vitamin D drops are not very expensive, typically about $6 for a 50-day supply, if one looks carefully. A 1-year supply of vitamin D drops would be about $40 to $50. Although this is not very much, we need to figure out how to make sure that everyone has access to vitamin D drops, including those who have limited financial resources.

Now at this point, one might ask if it would be best to simply forget about giving breast-fed babies vitamin D and just give extra vitamin D to the mother. This is not an unreasonable suggestion. However, it appears that a fairly large amount of vitamin D would be needed to be taken by mothers every day to achieve 300 to 400 IU per day of vitamin D in their milk. The amount needed, about 6000 IU per day, is above the currently established upper limit for vitamin D of 4000 IU per day (Wagner et al. 2006). However, it is likely that the risk of toxicity is relatively low in an individual mother. So, although we need much more safety and efficacy information about this approach before it can be widely advocated, it remains an option for selected mothers. Certainly, if a mother told us that she would not give her baby vitamin D, we would explain to her the option of taking high-dose vitamin D herself. Overall, the idea of dosing mother instead of baby is one that deserves much more research. This should be done in trials involving thousands of women to ensure safety, to understand compliance and tolerance, and most importantly, to identify the effects of different maternal supplementation levels on maternal milk vitamin D concentrations.

To summarize, there is compelling evidence that severe vitamin D deficiency leads to a markedly increased risk of the disease rickets. Rickets causes leg bowing and many other health problems. Vitamin D drops should be given to all breast-fed infants, and we should find a way to make this affordable for everyone. This recommendation does not depend on location. It is appropriate to give vitamin D drops to breast-fed infants throughout the world.

Calcium and Bone Minerals from Intravenous Nutrition

The management of bone mineral nutrition in infants and children who are being fed intravenously is an extremely specialized area of nutrition. However, some principles of management are important to understand and are worth consideration here. Let us focus specifically on how to provide enough calcium and phosphorus to meet the bone mineral needs of very low birth weight (VLBW), babies born at < 1500 grams birth weight (Prestridge et al. 1993).

Infants born this small must gradually learn how to tolerate feedings first from a tube into their stomach, and then directly from the breast or from a bottle. Their stomachs are tiny and the amount of food they receive must slowly be increased over several days. Typically, it takes about 10 days for an infant who weighs about 3 pounds (1350 grams) at birth to reach a full amount of feedings by a tube and about 14 days or more for infants born at about 2 pounds (900 grams). Infants who are born extremely small, such as 600 grams birth weight (slightly more than 1 pound) often take even longer to reach full feeds.

During the time in which they are not on a full amount of feedings, virtually all VLBW infants in the United States and much of the world will receive most or all of their nutrition intravenously. This type of nutrition is called parenteral nutrition (PN), or sometimes, total parenteral nutrition (TPN). As the amount of feeds is slowly increased, then the amount of intravenous nutrition is slowly decreased.

There are a lot of challenges specific to bone minerals when providing calcium and phosphorus intravenously. First, recall that calcium and phosphorus come together to mineralize bone. Therefore, when put in an intravenous form together, there is a risk they will join together and cause crystals in the intravenous fluids. As such, when planning and mixing TPN for neonates, a major concern is preventing this crystallization from occurring. To do this, a form of calcium called calcium gluconate is added along with either sodium or potassium phosphate. Pediatric pharmacists use special solubility curves to make sure that the amount of these minerals added to the TPN does not cause the minerals to precipitate out of solution and form crystals in the TPN bag. Such crystals would risk clotting off the intravenous line and also causing damage to the veins.

In 2011, shortages of key components of TPN occurred in the United States forcing undesired limitations of these components, especially calcium and phosphorus. The real possibility that such shortages will become long-term and recurring is a tremendous concern to those caring for very small or otherwise high-risk infants whose lives depend on intravenous nutrition (Holcombe et al. 2011). Even when the minerals are available, shortages of other TPN components, such as cysteine can lead to an inability to add optimal amounts of calcium and phosphorus to TPN.

Another big concern is that calcium given intravenously poses a serious risk of damaging veins and arteries in which it is given. It is not safe to give calcium via an artery, and this is not done in infants. When given through a vein, there is a risk that if the needle comes out of the vein, called infiltration, the skin and tissue around the intravenous entry point in the body can become swollen and damaged. Sometimes the damage is so severe as to cause permanent scarring and needs evaluation and management by a plastic surgeon.

If those two problems were not enough, VLBW infants, especially the smallest of them, are at very great risk for having dangerously low blood levels of calcium (called *hypocalcemia*) or too high levels (called *hypercalcemia*). Although hypercalcemia is often discussed as a risk of vitamin D intoxication, in this case it is not due to that. Instead, it is related to the difficulty the smallest infants have of producing and regulating the hormones that normalize blood calcium levels and also of mineralizing their very tiny bones.

At best, when using an intravenous line that goes into the main veins of the body, called a central line, it is possible to provide VLBW infants with about two-thirds of the calcium and phosphorus they need relative to how much they would have gotten while still *in utero*. This is not ideal, but it is not too inadequate given the challenges we have described. In babies who have long-term health problems requiring limitations in the amount of nutrition they can receive intravenously, or whose lungs require that they receive steroids intravenously, it is even more difficult to achieve adequate bone mineralization. Rickets remains a real problem in such preterm infants even with the best of modern neonatal intensive care.

Managing TPN in small infants requires the dedicated and close management of neonatologists, pharmacists, nurses, and dietitians. Feeding babies intravenously and making them grow safely when they cannot yet eat is one of the greatest challenges in all of neonatology. Globally, developing strategies to provide TPN in developing countries that are safe and effective is one of the most important areas that we are involved with. It is a tremendous privilege for us to work with doctors in developing countries to design strategies to help small infants survive in settings where they might otherwise have died due to malnutrition.

Iron and Solid Foods

First, it is important to fully recognize that with the possible exceptions of iron and vitamin D, breast milk has every nutrient a healthy full-term baby needs for at least 6 months of life. Specifically, from a bone health perspective, it really does not make much difference exactly when solid foods are introduced.

Any solid foods given from 4 to 6 months provide a small amount of calcium compared to breast milk. In some developing countries, the use of weaning foods that contain high amounts of phytates might pose a problem by interfering with calcium absorption, but even this is unlikely to be a big problem from 4 to 6 months of age. It may, however, become a much bigger problem after weaning from breast milk. Therefore, the timing for introduction of solid foods is not really an issue primarily related to bone health.

In considering when to add solid foods to an infant's diet, we generally are focusing on the primarily or exclusively breast-fed infant. This is an unbelievably contentious issue. Essentially, all scientists and experts in this area agree that from birth to 4 months of age, infants who are born at full-term (37 weeks gestation or more), and who are not low birth weight (that is, who are born at a weight greater than 2500 grams which is about 5 pounds 8 ounces), need nothing but breast milk and vitamin D until they are a full 4 months of age. Almost everyone agrees that by 6 months of age there are a lot of good reasons to begin breast-fed infants on solid foods and make sure they have a source of iron either from their solid foods *or* from an iron-containing vitamin source. For sure, there are some who argue that 6 months is too early for some babies, but few seriously doubt that most infants are ready for solid foods after 6 months of age, and therefore need some nonbreast milk iron source.

So, the battle—and it *is* a battle—is mostly about babies from 4 to 6 months of age. First, let us touch on the iron issue. In deciding when breast-fed babies need iron, one has to reconcile competing, confusing, complicated, and completely inadequate science. Let us call that the "4 C's" of scientific data.

The 4 C's of Scientific Data:

1. Is it Compelling?
2. Is it Confusing?
3. Is it Complicated?
4. Is it Completely inadequate?

Babies get their iron in the first 6 months of life almost entirely from the iron they have stored in their liver, their bone marrow, and their circulation *in utero*. Babies increase their blood volume such that they need about 0.75 to 1 mg daily of *new* iron to make the new red blood cells in their body. Breast milk consistently contains about 0.20 mg of iron in one day's supply. So, even though it is pretty well-absorbed (at most about 50%, but usually about 20%), it can, at best, provide about 0.10 mg of iron each day. So, most of babies' iron comes from what they can store before or at birth (Griffin and Abrams 2001; Abrams et al. 1997).

Not surprisingly, there is a huge variation in this among babies. This variation is related to a lot of factors, of which the most important include the baby's size, the mother's iron status, and how and when the umbilical cord was cut at birth. Organizations making public policy now need to take into account the large variation in these factors to protect infants from the consequences of anemia and low iron. Of course, there will be huge differences of opinion in how to do that.

Some groups (Fewtrell et al. 2010), have argued that beginning iron-containing solid foods at 4 months of age (or between 4 and 6 months) is likely to prevent the majority of babies from becoming iron deficient (Baker and Greer 2010; CDC 1998). In general, these groups argue that adding iron earlier is safe, that there is a small amount of research showing it leads to better outcomes in childhood, and that it is not difficult to do practically, among other reasons, because it just means adding iron to the vitamin D–containing drops babies are already getting.

Conversely other groups, including the World Health Organization (2002) and the Academy on Breastfeeding Medicine (2008), have argued that iron should not be started until 6 months of age along with solid foods. They and others consider that approaches including delayed cord clamping should be used, that high-risk infants can be individually monitored, and that limited research suggests some possible harmful effects of adding iron before 6 months of age. They also argue that adding iron in a drop before 6 months of age would discourage breast-feeding.

So, where does the truth lie? Well, as with so many issues, we have limited data, and it is hard to sort out. It is our view that no solids until 6 months is ideal and should be the standard of care that is recommended by dietitians and physicians caring for infants. However, as with many pediatric guidelines, this is not one that needs to be set out as a "do this or you're a bad parent" ideal. Rather it is something that each parent should discuss with their pediatric caregiver and given the equipoise in current science about the issue, come to their own conclusion. Thus, a parent does not need to feel guilty if their 5-month-old eats a jar of cereal, a few bites of pureed meat, or prepared infant meat products. Also, they should not be excessively concerned if a 6- or even 7-month-old breast-fed infant decides that the jar of baby food is not for them. Patience and persistence when introducing solid foods is all that is needed.

Well-meaning folks can easily look at this type of issue and come to very different conclusions. We think the data lean towards adding iron drops as recommended by the AAP sooner rather than later (i.e., at 4 months of age). Breast-fed infants should be getting vitamin D throughout this time period so at 4 months it is hardly a revolutionary change to simply switch to drops that also include iron. Many of these babies get some of their milk from a bottle, so it can be added to that if a caregiver does not want to squirt the drops into the baby's mouth. In general, the data showing negative effects on growth and infection are extremely limited and the potential of harm from low iron status is a more valid concern.

Knowing when to start solid foods and what nutrients are important for this age is key to figuring out what foods to feed your child. A somewhat common practice is to add cereal to bottles. The AAP recommends against this practice because it can cause children delays in developing skills needed for feeding themselves, it may displace important nutrients from breast milk, and it may contribute to overfeeding or overeating and obesity in the future. Babies spit up and sometimes spit up a lot. If the baby is growing and otherwise not upset by this, rarely is an intervention such as rice cereal needed. If an infant is becoming very upset frequently by spitting up, or if their growth is poor, then the pediatrician should consider a range of options, including the use of cereal. This should not be routine, however, and needs careful discussion with a pediatrician before being implemented.

Breast-Feeding and Nutrition for Infants in the Bible and Ancient Times

Ancient writings also covered the need for good nutrition in order for mothers to be able to breast-feed. The following passage comes from the Jewish writings called the Talmud.

> A nursing woman should not eat bad things while she is nursing him. What are these? Rav Kahana said: For instance, k'shut (a reddish clay), sprouts of grain, small fish and earth. Abaye said: Even pumpkins and quinces. Rav Papa said: Even a hearts

of palm and unripe dates. Rav Ashi said: Even kamka (a sauce with milk in it) and fish-hash. Some of these cause the flow of milk to stop while others cause the milk to become thick. (B. Ketubot 60b)

Obviously, the diet of Babylonian women 1700 years ago was quite different from our diet today. The second century Greek physician, Soranus, also provided details of the appropriate diet for nursing women.

A wet nurse ought to forgo leek and onions, garlic, preserved meat or fish, radish, and all preserved food and most vegetables because they are watery and not nourishing. Rather, she should partake of pure bread, egg yolk, brain, thrushes, the young of pigeons and domestic birds, rock fish, bass and suckling pig meat.

Paternal attitudes toward nursing were a factor in its success in ancient days, as they are today. This is a passage from the Talmud.

If the mother says that she wishes to nurse her child and the father does not want her to nurse it, we listen to her, because the suffering would be hers. What should be done when he says that she shall nurse the child and she says that she will not nurse it? Whenever nursing by the mother is not the practice of her family, we listen to her. (B. Ketubot 61a)

The Jewish sages suggest that forcing a mother to stop nursing would cause her to suffer. This presumably refers to both the physical discomfort of rapid weaning and the emotional suffering of a mother forcibly separated from her infant. However, if a woman comes from a wealthy family that usually hired wet nurses, this custom is followed. Here we see a great deal of sensitivity of the ancient writers in respecting a woman's wishes and family customs with regard to this very important aspect of mothering.

Another interesting reference to wet nurses from the Bible is found in the second chapter of Exodus in which the infant Moses is found in the river by the Pharaoh's daughter.

Then his sister asked Pharaoh's daughter, "Shall I go and get one of the Hebrew women to nurse the baby for you?" "Yes, go," she answered. So the girl went and got the baby's mother. Pharaoh's daughter said to her, "Take this baby and nurse him for me, and I will pay you." So the woman took the baby and nursed him. When the child grew older, she took him to Pharaoh's daughter and he became her son. She named him Moses, saying, "I drew him out of the water." Exodus 2:7-10 (New International Version)

The use of a wet-nurse was obviously considered culturally acceptable and was, therefore, quite common among women who could not breast-feed. While we know that Moses was three months old when the Pharaoh's daughter found him (Exodus 2:2), it is not clear how old he was when his mother weaned him.

There is considerable discussion in ancient Jewish literature regarding how long an infant should be nursed. This had important ramifications for the status of the infant, the mother, and the family unit. The following passages illustrate some of that discussion and even disagreement.

> A child should be nursed continuously for twenty-four months. From that age onward the child is to be regarded as one who sucks an abominable thing: these are the words of Rabbi Eliezer. And Rabbi Joshua says: the child may be breast-fed even for five years continuously. If he ceased after twenty-four months and started [being breast-fed] again he is to be regarded as sucking an abominable thing. (T. Niddah 2:3)

Jewish law (*halakhah*) follows Rabbi Joshua's words: a child should be nursed for two years and weaned by four years of age if healthy; five years of age if sickly. During the first two years of life, a child is allowed to resume nursing after having stopped for a time, but after two years of age, once the child is fully weaned, it does not return to being nursed. It is of note that some people today would consider breast-feeding a child after 24 months of age as inappropriate parenting. However, the AAP and many other organizations advocate for child-led weaning and do not set any given age by which weaning must occur.

Those of you who might be interested in reading more about ancient nutrition as it relates to pediatrics are welcome to read this book, *Jewish Parenting: Rabbinic Insights*, about it (Abrams and Abrams 1994).

References

Abrams SA. 2007. In utero physiology: Role in nutrient delivery and fetal development for calcium, phosphorus, and vitamin D. *Am J Clin Nutr* 85:604S–7S. A review of what happens before birth and some discussion about premature infants. (Free online.)

Abrams JZ and Abrams SA. 1994. *Jewish Parenting: Rabbinic Insights*. Lanham, MD: Jason Aronson Publishers, Inc. Not free but really inexpensive on Amazon.com and similar sites, http://www.amazon.com/gp/offer-listing/1568211759/ref=dp_olp_used?ie=UTF8&condition=used. (25 cents. What a deal! Of course, it is $3.99 for shipping.)

Abrams SA, Wen J, and Stuff JE. 1997. Absorption of calcium, zinc and iron from breast milk by 5- to 7-month-old infants. *Pediatr Res* 41:384–90. Generally absorption of iron in breast milk ranges from 20% to 40% in infants. This does not provide most of an infant's requirements for making new red blood cells. That must come from storage in the liver and other places, and later in infancy from additional dietary sources. (Not free online.)

Academy of Breastfeeding Medicine Board of Directors. 2008. ABM Statements: Position on breastfeeding. *Breastfeeding Medicine* 3:267–70. This is a fairly detailed statement related to supporting breast-feeding. (Free online.)

Baker RD, Greer FR, and the Committee on Nutrition of the American Academy of Pediatrics. 2010. Diagnosis and prevention of iron deficiency and iron-deficiency anemia in infants and young children (0–3 years of age). *Pediatrics* 126:1040–50. This report recommends providing breast-fed infants with some additional iron beginning at 4 months of age. This recommendation is potentially in conflict with the World Health Organization (WHO) on this issue as they recommend 6 months.

Bronner F, Salle BL, Putet G, Rigo J, and Senterre J. 1992. Net calcium absorption in premature infants: Results of 103 metabolic balance studies. *Am J Clin Nutr* 56:1037–44. This is an older study suggesting that vitamin D is not involved in calcium absorption in preterm infants. The real problem is that this hypothesis is almost impossible to test. It is not easier to test in full-term infants either. There just is not any good way to do multiple calcium absorption studies in the first weeks of life safely and without hurting the infants excessively (with multiple blood draws). Some important questions can be nearly impossible to answer. (Free online.)

Centers for Disease Control (CDC): Recommendations to Prevent and Control Iron Deficiency in the United States. 1998. *MMWR* 47(RR-3);1–36, http://wonder.cdc.gov/wonder/prevguid/m0051880/m0051880.asp. This is the classic CDC statement about iron. It has not been revised to date by the CDC. (Free online.)

Craviari T, Pettifor JM, Thacher TD, Meisner C, Arnaud J, and Fischer PR. 2008. Rickets Convergence Group. Rickets: An Overview and Future Directions, with Special Reference to Bangladesh. A summary of the Rickets Convergence Group meeting, Dhaka, 26–27 January 2006. *J Health Popul Nutr* 26:112–21. A great review article with a lot of images of rickets that are of value in understanding the condition. Focuses on global rickets. (Free online.)

Fewtrell M, Wilson DC, Booth I, and Lucas A. 2010. Six months of exclusive breast feeding: How good is the evidence? *BMJ* 342:c5955, doi: 10.1136/bmj.c5955. This set off a firestorm of controversy and letters to the editors. Note that the authors did not argue against breast-feeding, only that it might be a good idea to start solid foods a bit earlier than 6 months. Many, but not all, online respondents disagreed. We tend to support the WHO position of waiting until 6 months to start solids and only giving iron and vitamin D drops before then. The evidence just is not there to be sure and probably never will be. Families need to use their best judgment on this along with the views of their pediatric caregiver. (Not free online.)

Fudge NJ and Kovacs CS. 2010. Pregnancy up-regulates intestinal calcium absorption and skeletal mineralization independently of the vitamin D receptor. *Endocrinology* 151:886–95. This concerns animal research data suggesting that the increase in calcium absorption during pregnancy is not related primarily to vitamin D. (Free online.)

Griffin IJ and Abrams SA. 2001. Iron and breastfeeding. *Pediatr Clin N Amer* 48:401–13. This is a review of the physiology associated with iron and breastfeeding. (Not free online.)

Holcombe B, Andris DA, Brooks G, Houston DR, and Plogsted SW. 2011. Parenteral nutrition electrolyte/mineral product shortage considerations. *JPEN J Parenter Enteral Nutr* 35:434–6. (Not free online, but the American Society for Parenteral and Enteral Nutrition [A.S.P.E.N.] and the FDA maintain Web sites describing known shortages such as http://www.nutritioncare.org/News/ PN_Electrolyte_Shortage_Update/. More information would be helpful.)

Institute of Medicine. 2011. Dietary Reference Intakes for Calcium and vitamin D. Washington, DC: National Academy Press. See annotation in Chapter 2 "References."

Jarjou LM, Prentice A, Sawo Y, Laskey MA, Bennett J, Goldberg GR, and Cole TJ. 2006. Randomized, placebo-controlled, calcium supplementation study in pregnant Gambian women: Effects on breast milk calcium concentrations and infant birth weight, growth, and bone mineral accretion in the first year of life. *Am J Clin Nutr* 83:657–66. This is a fascinating study of women in the Gambia with very low calcium intakes and low breast milk calcium in whom high-dose calcium supplements changed little if anything. (Free online.)

Mitchell SM, Rogers SP, Hicks PD, Hawthorne KM, Parker BR, and Abrams SA. 2009. High frequencies of elevated alkaline phosphatase activity and rickets exist in extremely low birth weight infants despite current nutritional support. *BMC Pediatr* 9:47. This is a review of the problem of rickets in preterm infants including a clinically usable flowsheet for how to evaluate very small infants in the neonatal ICU setting. (Free online.)

Ozkan B. 2010. Nutritional rickets. *J Clin Res Pediatr Endocrinol* 2:137–43. E-pub November 1, 2010. This is another review paper with X-rays that is helpful in understanding the condition. (Free online.)

Perrine CG, Sharma AJ, Jefferds ME, Serdula MK, and Scanlon KS. 2010. Adherence to vitamin D recommendations among U.S. infants. *Pediatrics* 125:627–32. Mothers do not give their babies the recommended amounts of vitamin D. Why? We think a lot is due to cost and lack of education about the importance of vitamin D for breast-fed infants. (Free online.)

Prestridge LL, Schanler RJ, Shulman RJ, Burns PA, and Laine LL. 1993. Effect of parenteral calcium and phosphorus therapy on mineral retention and bone mineral content in very–low–birth–weight infants. *J Pediatr* 122:761–8. An oldie but goodie that explains how to get more minerals into intravenous nutrition for premature infants. (Not free online.)

Rigo J, Pieltain C, Salle B, Senterre J. and Enteral C. 2007. Calcium, phosphate and vitamin D requirements and bone mineralization in preterm infants. *Acta Paediatr* 96:969–74. The European view is a little different than the U.S. one. In general, the Europeans target a somewhat lower calcium and phosphorus intake in preterm infants and a higher vitamin D intake. There are no direct comparisons available. (Not free online.)

Swinburne LM. 2006. Rickets and the Fairfax family receipt books. *J R Soc Med* 99:3915. This is an incredible history of rickets providing accounts dating it to the earliest part of the 17th century. (Not free online.)

Thacher TD, Fischer PR, and Pettifor JM. 2007. Rickets: Vitamin D and calcium deficiency. *J Bone Miner Res* 22: 638. A fascinating letter to the editor that discusses the possibility that wet nursing was related to rickets in the 17th century. The suggestion is that it was related to calcium in milk, not vitamin D. However, there is not much evidence to support this idea. Still it is as legitimate a hypothesis as many other historical ones of this sort. (Free online.)

Wagner CL, Hulsey TC, Fanning D, Ebeling M, and Hollis BW. 2006. High-dose vitamin D_3 supplementation in a cohort of breast-feeding mothers and their infants: A 6-month follow-up pilot study. *Breastfeed Med* 1:59–70. This is one way to get enough vitamin D into infants. It would be nice to see much larger studies related to both safety and efficacy of this approach. But, giving high-dose vitamin D to mothers instead of dosing breast-feeding infants is an option for those who wish to consider it. (Not free online via the publisher, but appears to be available from other resources online.)

Wagner CL, Greer FR, and American Academy of Pediatrics, Section on Breastfeeding and Committee on Nutrition. 2008. Prevention of rickets and vitamin D deficiency in infants, children, and adolescents. *Pediatrics.* 122(5):1142–52. [Published correction appears in 2009 *Pediatrics* 123(1):197.] See annotation in Chapter 2 "References." (Free online.)

World Health Organization. 2002. Nutrient Adequacy of Exclusive Breastfeeding for the Term Infant during the First Six Months of Life. Geneva, Switzerland: World Health Organization. http://www.who.int/nutrition/topics/exclusive_breastfeeding/en/index.html. This is the WHO position related to delaying the introduction of solid foods until 6 months of age. Not everyone agrees with the WHO on this, but it is generally the currently accepted perspective throughout the world. (Free online.)

chapter four

Toddlers (children younger than 4 years of age)

Toddlers, whom we will define here as children 12 to 48 months of age, are the great black hole of nutritional research. Almost no one does research on this age group! Why? Well, anyone who has had a toddler, has sat next to a toddler on an airplane, or who remembers being a toddler will know the answer to this one. Nutritional research involves getting good diet histories, drawing blood, and collecting urine and stool samples. This is not exactly the easiest thing to do with the average 2-year-old. Actually, this is pretty hard to do with teens and adults too, but it is easier to distract them.

Because of these challenges, we have the least amount of information about the nutritional requirements of this age group. For many years, most dietary guidelines for toddlers were derived either from *guessing up* or *rounding down*. That is, either data from infants were increased based on the greater body weight of toddlers, or data in older children were decreased based on the smaller body weight of toddlers. It is not surprising that this is not a very accurate approach. The diets and bodies of toddlers are not well approximated by infants or by older children.

Specific to bone health, we know from some fairly extensive studies measuring bone mineralization in toddlers done with Dual-Energy X-ray Absorptiometry (DXA), that bone growth is relatively slow in this age group. It is a bit slower than in babies or in older children. Also, it is not the easiest thing in the world to get a toddler to be still long enough for the 2 minutes it takes to do a DXA scan, but it is possible. And with the help of trained and patient technicians, nurses, dietitians, and mothers, it can be done (Figure 4.1). Nonetheless, we know extremely little about optimal nutrition for toddlers or what to do about the common decrease in appetite that occurs around 2 years of age.

Calcium and the recommended dietary allowance (RDA)

Toddlers who have a typical diet including 2 servings each day of dairy products are likely to meet their daily requirement for calcium of 700 mg per day (IOM 2011) readily. Even one serving of dairy with another

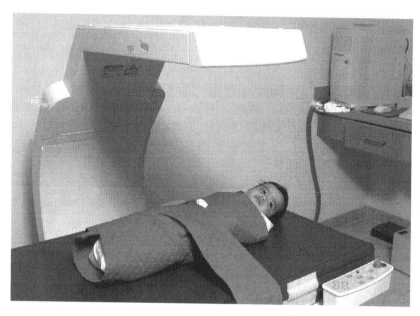

Figure 4.1 Small child getting a DXA bone scan. The radiation exposure from a DXA scan is extremely small, comparable to that received during usual activities such as going to the beach. Photo courtesy of Robert and Penni Hicks and Adam Gillum.

serving of fortified juice should do the trick to reach about 700 mg/day (Lynch et al. 2007).

Note that the 700 mg per day is a Recommended Dietary Allowance (RDA). As we begin to talk about children after infancy, we now have two new dietary terms to look at in addition to the Adequate Intake (AI) used for infants. These two terms are the Estimated Average Requirement (EAR) and the RDA. Definitions of these terms are found in Chapter 2. A full-length book explanation of all of these terms is found at the IOM website at http://books.nap.edu/openbook.php?record_id=9956. This can be downloaded page-by-page free online or purchased.

What do these terms really mean in common usage? The EAR is an average requirement meant to meet the needs of about half the population. That is, if a child consumes a diet providing the EAR for calcium, then, based on the average bioavailability of the calcium, they will have a 50% chance of meeting their needs, or in this case, of having a typical and appropriate increase in bone growth. This sounds reasonable, but most people do not want to have a 50% chance of meeting their dietary needs, they want a 100% chance.

However, a 100% chance of meeting dietary needs is not something we might really want. If we tell everyone to take in so much calcium in order to be certain that even those who have the worst calcium bioavail-ability will meet their needs, then we will undoubtedly be making some individuals toxic or at least approaching an absorbed amount that might be problematic. That is, there is a trade-off between ensuring the unusu-ally high needs of some are met, and making sure those high needs do not get translated into policies that would make a lot of other people toxic.

To resolve this problem, the nutrition community has always ensured that individuals who wish to be virtually certain of meeting their dietary needs have an intake that would meet the needs about 97.5% of the pop-ulation. This intake is called the *RDA*. Now, the most obvious question is "Where did they come up with the 97.5 percentile"? That number is 2 standard deviations above the mean. This is a value used for almost everything in terms of nutrition. For example, the current World Health Organization (WHO) growth curves mark overweight and underweight lines at the 3rd and 97th percentiles respectively, which is two standard deviations below and above the average (Grummer-Strawn, Reinhold, and Krebs 2010; WHO 2006). For some uses, people may look at three stan-dard deviations, slightly above the 99 percentile. But for most nutrition purposes, the trade-off between safety and toxicity has been set at 2 stan-dard deviations above the mean or about the 97th percentile.

What are some of the implications of these numbers? Well, one is that we should be cautious about saying something like "Your child has a cal-cium intake of 690 mg per day which is inadequate for him." We discussed this issue in Chapter 2. This type of analysis is untrue and misleading to boot! If the EAR for calcium is 500 mg per day then there is more than a 95% chance that the child is meeting their nutritional needs for calcium with an intake of 690 mg per day. Since dietary intake measurements are never that accurate (see discussion in Chapter 2), and diets are never that consistent on a day-to-day basis, we should avoid using strict cutoffs to define inadequacy anyway.

The bottom line is that the RDA can give individuals a general target for their dietary intake that will *almost* certainly be enough. That does not mean that an intake below the RDA is *not enough* though, or that there is an individual or community crisis when someone does not meet the RDA. Mathematically, we can calculate the likely proportion of people who are deficient if we know the average, the distribution of intakes, and have an EAR and RDA. This is important for dietary planning, but less so for indi-vidual counseling and guidance. In this method (http://www.nap.edu/openbook.php?record_id=9956&page=208), the proportion of individuals with intakes below the EAR is the proportion of the population that is deficient (Barr 2006). Take a look at Table 4.1 through Table 4.4 for an idea of usual intakes and the proportion of individuals below the EAR for cal-cium and vitamin D.

Table **4.1** Nutrient Intakes from Food: Mean
Amounts Consumed per Individual, by Gender and
Age, in the United States, 2007–2008

Gender and Age (years)	Vitamin D (IU)	Calcium (mg)
Males:		
2–5	260	1009
6–11	220	1034
12–19	236	1173
Females:		
2–5	244	957
6–11	184	885
12–19	152	878

Source: NHANES 2007–2008, *What We Eat in America,
Individuals 2 Years and Over (Excluding Breast-Fed Children)
Day 1 Dietary Intake Data, Weighted,* Washington, DC: U.S.
Department of Agriculture, (Revised August 2010).

Table **4.2** How Many Toddlers Do Not Get Enough Calcium?

Life Stage Group	RDA (mg/day)	EAR (mg/day)	Mean Values of Estimated Intakes (mg/day)	% Below EAR
Males: 1–3 years old	700	500	998	5%
Females: 1–3 years old	700	500	986	4%

Source: NHANES 2005–2006, Calcium (mg/day): Percent of EAR Consumed in the United
States from Food Sources Only Based on Mean Values of Estimated Intake.

What do children eat?

Thanks to national surveys such as "What We Eat in America" (http://
www.ars.usda.gov/Services/docs.htm?docid=13793), a part of the National
Health and Nutrition Examination Survey (NHANES), we have a reasonable idea of what children in the United States eat, and we can figure out
how many children do not have enough dietary calcium and vitamin D.
Only about 5% of 1- to 3-year-old children have intakes below the EAR for
calcium. That means we clearly know that only about 5% of 1- to 3-year-
old children are not getting enough calcium in their diets. This is great
news. The picture for vitamin D is not so great, but we will get to that in
a moment.

Let's go back to calcium and toddlers. The average U.S. intake of calcium for boys is 970 mg per day, and the RDA of 700 mg per day falls at

Table 4.3 How Many Toddlers Do Not Get Enough Vitamin D?

Life Stage Group	RDA (IU/day)	EAR (IU/day)	Mean Values of Estimated Intakes (IU/day)	% Below EAR
Males: 1–3 years old	600	400	288	76%
Females: 1–3 years old	600	400	272	82%

Source: NHANES 2005–2006, Vitamin D (IU/day): Percent of EAR Consumed in the United States from Food Sources Only Based on Mean Values of Estimated Intake.

Table 4.4 How Many Toddlers Do Not Get Enough Vitamin D Even When Considering Intake from Supplements?

Life Stage Group	RDA (IU/day)	EAR (IU/day)	Mean Values of Estimated Intakes (IU/day)	% Below EAR
Males: 1–3 years old	600	400	364	61%
Females: 1–3 years old	600	400	336	71%

Source: Bailey RL, Dodd KW, Goldman JA, Gahche JJ, Dwyer JT, Moshfegh AJ, Sempos CT, and Picciano MF, 2010, Estimation of Total Usual Calcium and Vitamin D Intake in the United States, *Journal of Nutrition,* "Appendix H."

about the 20% percentile of intake (IOM 2011 "Appendix H"). The numbers for girls are virtually identical with an average intake of 940 mg per day and 700 mg per day at about the 15th percentile of intake. Therefore, when counseling an individual in this age group, about 15% to 20% will be below the RDA and about 4% to 5% below the EAR (Table 4.2). On the whole, it should not be too hard to get intakes up to about 700 mg per day for most children in this age group who have some dairy intake. In terms of population deficiencies though, it is clear that we are mostly doing okay in this age group, with only 4% to 5% below the EAR and, therefore, that is the proportion of the population that is defined as being deficient.

Vitamin D

The situation with vitamin D in the toddler age group is more complicated and one in which we have very little data. The new dietary guidelines (DRI values) provide an EAR of 400 IU per day and an RDA of 600 IU per day. These are the values for all age groups from 1 to 70 years of age. The vitamin D needs of toddlers are complex. On one hand, since toddlers are smaller than older children or adults, they should need somewhat less vitamin D to achieve the targeted serum vitamin D levels. The target serum 25(OH)D is 20 ng/mL for the RDA and most of them will achieve this level with 600 IU per day intake (IOM 2011).

The pediatric data available at the time of the IOM report indicated that the response of serum 25(OH)D to vitamin D supplementation was very similar in children from about 6 years of age through adulthood. There were no data for toddlers at the time of the IOM report. Therefore, the IOM committee decided to be cautious and use the same 600 IU per day value for toddlers to make sure that they had adequate vitamin D to reach the targeted serum levels of 25(OH)D. Furthermore, had the RDA been set lower in this age group, for example at 400 IU per day, that would have meant an EAR < 400 IU per day. This might have caused some real confusion considering the previous AI of 400 IU per day for infants and children and the current AI of 400 IU per day for infants. It might have implied that vitamin D requirements went down after a year of age, which would not be true.

Rickets in toddlers

Beyond vitamin D in toddlers, there is also the concern about the risk of rickets in this age group. As we discussed with infants, the problem is making sure that the skeleton receives the 80 to 100 mg per day of calcium that is needed for adequate bone mineralization. In the majority of toddlers, a calcium intake of at least 500 mg per day will lead to this amount being retained by the skeleton. Absorption of calcium is lower from cow's milk and from other sources than it is from breast milk. Only 30% to 40% may be absorbed. Still, there is a reasonable margin of safety.

Several situations may pose special risk though. One is for toddlers who do not drink cow's milk or other calcium and vitamin D-fortified beverages. These may be infants who are still receiving their milk via breast-feeding in the second year of life without receiving vitamin supplementation or those who are simply not given virtually any milk, dairy products, or other vitamin D-fortified beverages. This situation is common in many resource-poor countries including much of Africa. The other situation is children who have diets with high levels of inhibitors of calcium absorption, such as toddlers in developing countries. They often have little, if any, dairy products in their daily diet, and they eat lots of foods containing substances that inhibit calcium absorption, such as phytates. Phytates are mostly found in some whole grain products such as cereals and breads and they can hinder the amount of calcium that is absorbed by the body. In a usual diet, this does not cause any problem, but it can be a problem in societies with very little dairy and lots of whole grains in the diet.

How to achieve vitamin D intakes in toddlers

Recognizing that 600 IU per day RDA is the target for dietary intake with a bit of a safety margin for those children with minimal dairy in their diet, how do we get to this level in the diet of a toddler? This is not too easy to do on just their usual diet.

One approach is to increase dairy intake, but it would be difficult to get 600 IU of vitamin D daily *only* from milk in a child this age this way, and there is a possible concern that drinking a liter or more of milk each day may be harmful for toddlers because it may lead to poor iron status (http://pediatrics.about.com/od/weeklyquestion/a/04_toomuch_milk. htm). There are some older infants and toddlers who drink huge amounts of milk each day. Although the reasons remain somewhat unclear, drinking very large quantities of milk is associated with a worse iron status in older infants and toddlers. Reasons may be related to the loss of small amounts of blood in the stool from excessive milk drinking, although this has not been convincingly demonstrated. In general, 2 to 3 servings of dairy each day, providing 200 to 300 IU of vitamin D daily is appropriate and a good practice in this age group. In addition to milk, fortified foods can offer additional vitamin D in a toddler's diet.

If the toddler had been on a multivitamin with iron supplement as an infant, one thing to do would be to continue it during the second year of life and perhaps to transition to a chewable one when the child was ready for that. Most multivitamins for children contain 400 IU of vitamin D allowing a child to reach 600 IU readily when combined with diet.

The bottom line is that for toddlers, diet is currently a challenging way to get to a full 600 IU per day of vitamin D. This may change as more foods become fortified, but, for now, it would be difficult. Currently, the 50th percentile of all vitamin D intake (including supplements) for children is 330 IU per day for boys and 300 IU/day for girls. The RDA of 600 IU per day is at about the 80th percentile for boys and the 90th percentile for girls. If one excludes supplement use, then 600 IU per day is close to the 97 to 99th percentile for boys and girls (Table 4.3). In other words, only approximately 1% to 3% of toddlers reach a vitamin D intake of 600 IU per day from their diet alone. Using the EAR method to determine deficiency, over half of toddlers have a deficient intake from diet and supplements although this calculation is imprecise due to the variable effects of sunshine exposure.

Some common sources of calcium and vitamin D are shown in Table 4.5. To reach 600 IU per day just from milk for example, would require a milk intake of 48 ounces, a value well above the amount that would be recommended or generally observed as a milk intake in toddlers.

Table 4.5 Common Sources of Calcium and Vitamin D

Food	Serving	Calcium (mg)	Vitamin D (IU)
Cod Liver Oil	1 tbsp	0	1360
Salmon (cooked)	3 oz	10	795
Mushrooms exposed to ultraviolet (UV) light (portabella, raw)	1 cup	0	400
Milk—with added calcium, vitamins A & D	8 fl oz	300	100
Orange Juice—with added calcium & vitamin D	8 fl oz	350	100
Soymilk—with added calcium, vitamins A & D	8 fl oz	280	100
Tuna fish (canned in oil)	3 oz	10	200
Sardines (canned in oil)	3 oz	325	164
Egg, whole	1 large	25	40
Yogurt—with added calcium & vitamin D	6 oz	200	40
Margarine—with added calcium & vitamin D	1 tbsp	100	40
Fortified ready-to-eat cereal	1 cup	100	20

Note: Calcium and vitamin D content of fortified products may vary between brands.

Other nutrients

Now that we are beyond infancy, it is time to consider further the role of some other nutrients in bone health in children. Amongst the most important are macronutrients, especially protein and omega-3 fatty acids, and micronutrients such as magnesium, zinc and phosphorus. We would like to consider these briefly here, remembering that they are important at any age.

First, let us start with protein. This was discussed briefly in Chapter 1 but will be reconsidered here. Protein is the building block, or more technically, the matrix, into which the bone minerals, calcium, and phosphorus are deposited to form normal bone. Protein deficiency leads to inadequate bone formation. Whether high protein intakes are harmful for bone, or whether the protein from meat is less beneficial than nonmeat protein for bone health, are sources of controversy in adults. In pediatrics, it can be said with some certainty that there is no evidence at all that normal healthy diets, including proteins from all sources (meat, dairy, and vegetable) cause any negative effects on bone.

Now let us turn to a hot topic: omega-3 fatty acids such as are found naturally in fish oil. Covering the potential health benefits of omega-3s for all ages would be beyond the scope of this book, but it is important to note that animal studies and increasing numbers of human studies show a small benefit for bone health as well as many other health benefits of omega-3s (Farina et al. 2011). The reason for the bone effect is not entirely certain, but there may be enhanced absorption for a small amount of minerals with a diet rich in omega-3s.

As far as micronutrients, the most important considerations for bone health are phosphorus, magnesium, and zinc. Important bone health nutrients also include vitamin K and the trace mineral boron, but these will not be covered here as there is very little data relating intakes of these nutrients to bone health in children. There are also interesting considerations related to excess sodium leading to high urinary calcium loss.

Phosphorus is a mineral that has gotten somewhat of a bad reputation because there is concern that high phosphorus intakes may inhibit calcium absorption. Certainly there is concern about the effects of high phosphorus intakes from soda on bone health. The reality is that the concern is probably greater than the actual effect. Phosphorus is a necessary component of the diet for bone health. Calcium must complex with phosphorus to mineralize bone. This occurs at about a 2:1 ratio (mg:mg) of calcium to phosphorus. However, whereas 99% of all of the calcium in the body is in bone, only 80% of the phosphorus is in bone. Therefore, it is possible to become phosphorus deficient during rapid bone growth, and this is common in premature infants as phosphorus serves *double duty*. Phosphorus absorption is partly controlled by vitamin D, so severe vitamin D deficiency can also decrease phosphorus absorption and worsen phosphorus deficiency.

In general, a typical diet in a child, that includes meat and dairy but limited phosphorus–containing sodas, is safe, effective, and healthy. Children who are vegans and avoid all meat and dairy may have more challenges in meeting their phosphorus requirements or may need a supplement, but this is not common among toddlers.

Magnesium and zinc are two very undervalued nutrients largely because of how little research has been done regarding them, especially in children. They have many health benefits throughout the life cycle: regulating blood pressure, enhancing growth, regulating appetite, and serving as a component of bone. In general, children's magnesium intakes are somewhat on the low side. Common sources of magnesium among children are nuts, whole grains, and peanut butter (Table 4.6). Zinc in the diet of children mostly comes from meats, seafood, eggs, and milk, or fortified foods such as cereals.

Magnesium absorption is not significantly controlled by vitamin D. However, there is some concern that high amounts of calcium without adequate magnesium can be harmful, especially in adults, although the evidence for this is still being investigated, and there are no data on this issue in children. Zinc absorption is not regulated by vitamin D, but zinc is an absolutely crucial and very underappreciated nutrient. It is a component of healthy bone. Furthermore, zinc deficiency decreases appetite and

Table 4.6 Common Food Sources of Magnesium (mg per serving)

Food	Serving	Magnesium (mg)
Halibut (cooked)	3 oz	90
Almonds	1 oz	80
Cashews	1 oz	75
Spinach (cooked)	½ cup	75
Fortified ready-to-eat cereal	1 cup	40–100
Oatmeal (instant, fortified, prepared with water)	1 cup	55
Potato (baked with skin)	1 medium	50
Peanut butter (smooth)	2 tbsp	50
Yogurt (plain, skim milk)	8 oz	45
Baked Beans	½ cup	40
Chocolate Milk	1 cup	33
Banana (raw)	1 medium	30
Milk (2% reduced-fat)	1 cup	27
Raisins (seedless)	½ cup	25

Source: U.S. Department of Agriculture, Agricultural Research Service, 2003, U.S. Department of Agriculture (USDA) National Nutrient Database for Standard Reference, Release 16, *Nutrient Data Laboratory,* http://www.nal.usda.gov/fnic/foodcomp.

slows overall growth. It may make many infections worse, including common diarrheal illnesses and pneumonia. It may also make human immunodeficiency virus (HIV) infections worse. In developing countries, zinc deficiency is a major problem and one that has been challenging to solve. This relates largely to the difficulty of balancing iron and zinc in highly absorbable forms in the meals or supplements given to small children. When too much iron is given, especially in the form of supplements, then zinc status worsens in many populations. This is less of a concern in the United States where iron and zinc are primarily provided from diet rather than supplements.

Which Milk Should Toddlers Drink?

If we stretch things a bit and define toddlers as being from 9 months to 4 years of age, we have a lot of choices. Infants can be breast-fed with the recommendation being to breast-feed until 12 months of age or as long thereafter as mother and child wish. Many groups recommend some breast-feeding up to two years of age or longer. We can provide infant formulas, toddler formulas, whole cow's milk, low-fat cow's milk, skim cow's milk, soymilk, ultra-heat treated (UHT) cow's milk, and a few others.

The traditional approach in the United States is to transition from either infant formula or breast-feeding to whole cow's milk at about one year of age. Sometimes families are very dogmatic on this. There is no need to pour the glass of regular milk at the first birthday party. Rather, it is best to gradually switch from infant formula at about 1 year of age over a period of a week or two. This is a good time to introduce cup feeding as well.

For breast-fed infants, child-directed weaning should be done gradually. There is no absolute age at which a child should be switched to cow's milk from breast-feeding or bottles of expressed breast milk.

One recent recommendation that is not widely known is that the AAP revised its recommendations for milk choice for children under 2 years of age. Prior to the revised recommendation it was commonly understood that only whole milk should be used. However, more recent recommendations (Daniels, Greer, and the Committee on Nutrition 2008) say that reduced-fat milk can by used for children 12 to 24 months or for whom overweight or obesity is a concern, or for those who have a family history of obesity, dyslipidemia (such as very high triglyceride or cholesterol levels), or cardiovascular disease. Usually it is 2% milk that is intended for use in this circumstance because milk fat remains important for brain development in the second year of life. After 2 years of age, the fat content of the diet for brain development does not need to be as high. Children can be transitioned to 1% or fat-free milk. Although everyone is different, most families will find that a slow decrease in fat content of milk from whole milk to fat-free milk, or skim milk (0.5% milk) over a period of time is well accepted by every member of the family.

Global Malnutrition in Infants and Small Children: A Bone Mineral Perspective

Over the last decade, we have made many international trips related to our research in mineral metabolism as well as growth and training in neonatal care (http://www.texaschildrens.org/Professionals/WHOCC.aspx). The high incidence of bone health related problems in developing countries is one important condition that may surprise people. These problems include rickets in infants and toddlers, and very low vitamin D and calcium levels in the blood of newborns leading to neonatal health problems.

One country with a high incidence of rickets is Nigeria. In some areas up to 10% of the children are affected. This appears to be primarily due to an extremely low intake of calcium among children there. Calcium intakes may often be about 150–200 mg per day, well below the recommended amounts for children over 1 year of age. We evaluated a number of different factors associated with the rickets and could not clearly identify a particular problem with other dietary components that was leading to the rickets (Thacher et al. 2009). It is likely that genetics, combined with the extremely low calcium intakes is the primary culprit. Vitamin D plays a small role in this, but overall "An optimal 25(OH)D level cannot be identified that will reliably prevent rickets, nor can one be found that causes the condition" among Nigerian children (Thacher and Abrams 2010).

Another country with a high incidence of what is in all likelihood primarily calcium–deficient rickets is Bangladesh (http://centre.icddrb.org/pub/publication.jsp?classificationID=56&pubID=10220). As many as about 1% of small children there have clinical rickets. In Bangladesh, this translates to at least tens of thousands of children. In the United States, there is concern over a few dozen cases of rickets. This pales in comparison with the situation in other countries.

In Bangladesh, Nigeria, and many other countries, further research is needed into the role of vitamin D, calcium, and other components including protein in the children's diet to best battle the high rate of rickets.

Is It Child Abuse, Is It Rickets, or Is It Something Else?

In recent years some intense disputes have developed over whether some cases that have been treated as child abuse (nonaccidental injury) are actually undiagnosed cases of rickets. This issue has been debated both in the medical literature and in the mass media.

It is impossible for us to go back and determine whether individual cases were misdiagnosed, or whether the system by which individual families were accused, investigated, and prosecuted was applied properly or fairly. However, we can comment a bit about this from a medical and dietary perspective.

First, infants can have *weak bones* either due to rickets or more general low bone mineral content of their bones. They may also have a rare condition called *osteogenesis imperfecta* (Pandya et al. 2011). Rickets in newborns is much more likely for babies born at less that 32 weeks gestation or less than about 4 pounds. It can also occur in infants who are exclusively breast-fed without vitamin D supplementation, and rarely it can occur in infants or older children with hormonal and metabolic diseases. Such infants are more likely to fracture their bones, and the fractures can appear similar sometimes to the types of fractures that typically occur with nonaccidental injury.

However, absent this type of history, the likelihood of multiple fractures of the bones in an infant or small child from rickets is low. A serum 25(OH)D level that is extremely low, combined with certain other blood testing, can help identify the child with mild or early rickets but it is only one piece of information. However, this situation should be uncommon and generally easily identified when combined with radiological findings.

We are not experts in nonaccidental injury and do not wish to comment on how it is evaluated and prosecuted. However, nonaccidental injury is a real problem, and finding a low serum 25(OH)D level is not enough to assume that such a case is actually due to rickets (Schilling et al. 2011). An expert radiologist should be consulted to evaluate X-rays of the wrists and knees to determine if rickets is present, and a comprehensive history, physical exam, and lab testing evaluation should be done to determine if rickets is likely as an etiology for multiple fractures. Evaluation for rare genetic causes of rickets or for possible osteogenesis imperfecta may be needed.

References

Barr SI. 2006. Applications of dietary reference intakes in dietary assessment and planning. *Appl Physiol Nutr Metab* 31:66–73. This is a summary article of how to use the DRI values. Similar information can be found at the IOM Web site as part of many of the reports related to the DRI guidelines and food policy. (Not free online.)

Daniels SD, Greer FR, and Committee on Nutrition. 2008. Lipid screening and cardiovascular health in childhood. *Pediatrics* 122:198–208. There are some very controversial opinions about screening high-risk children for lipid disorders

and for allowing lower-fat milk in small children in certain situations including obesity. The specific quote is, "For children between 12 months and 2
years of age for whom overweight or obesity is a concern or who have a family history of obesity, dyslipidemia, or [cardiovascular disease] CVD, the use
of reduced-fat milk would be appropriate." (Free online.)

Farina EK, Kiel DP, Roubenoff R, Schaefer EJ, Cupples LA, and Tucker KL. 2011.
Protective effects of fish intake and interactive effects of long-chain polyun-
saturated fatty acid intakes on bone mineral density at the hip in older adults:
The Framingham Osteoporosis Study. *Am J Clin Nutr* 93:1142–51. This is one
of several well-performed studies indicating a possible benefit of omega-3
fatty acids (fish oil) on bone health. (Free online in mid-2012.)

Grummer-Strawn LM, Reinold C, Krebs NF, and Centers for Disease Control
and Prevention (CDC). 2010. Use of WHO and CDC growth charts for
children aged 0–59 months in the United States. MMWR Recomm Rep.
September 10;59(RR-9);1–15. See more description of this issue in Chapter
12. (Free online.)

Institute of Medicine. 2011. *Dietary Reference Intakes for Calcium and vitamin D.*
Washington, DC: National Academy Press. See annotation in Chapter 2
"References."

Lynch MF, Griffin IJ, Hawthorne KM, Chen Z, Hamzo M, and Abrams SA. 2007.
Calcium balance in 1- to 4-year-old children. *Am J Clin Nutr.* 85:750–4. This is
the paper, for those interested in seeing the math for children, that describes
calcium balance in small children, and how it can be used to set dietary recommendations. (Free online.)

Pandya NK, Baldwin K, Kamath AF, Wenger DR, and Hosalkar HS. 2011.
Unexplained fractures: Child abuse or bone disease? A systematic review.
Clin Orthop Relat Res 469:805–12. This is a very important and profoundly
controversial topic. There are bone diseases and presentations that can be
confused with nonaccidental injury. We must learn more about making these
distinctions appropriately. (Free online.)

Schilling S, Wood JN, Levine MA, Langdon D, and Christian CW. 2011. Vitamin D
status in abused and nonabused children younger than 2 years old with fractures. *Pediatrics* 127:835–41. The concluding sentences say it all: "Suboptimal
vitamin D status was not associated with a diagnosis of abuse or the presence of multiple fractures or rib or metaphyseal fractures, suggesting that
a strong association between vitamin D insufficiency and fracture types
related to abuse is unlikely. Our findings indicate that a low serum 25(OH)
D should not discourage consideration of abuse when a child presents with
unexplained fractures." (Not free online.)

Thacher TD and Abrams SA. 2010. Relationship of calcium absorption with 25(OH)
D and calcium intake in children with rickets. *Nutr Rev* 68:682–8. Usually,
rickets in Africa is not primarily caused by vitamin D deficiency, and calcium
absorption in this population is not closely linked to serum 25(OH)D. (Not
free online.)

Thacher TD, Aliu O, Griffin IJ, Pam SD, O'Brien KO, Imade GE, and Abrams
SA. 2009. Meals and dephytinization affect calcium and zinc absorption in
Nigerian children with rickets. J Nutr 139:926–32. Removing the phytates
from a typical Nigerian meal improved zinc absorption but had little effect
on calcium absorption in small children. Overall, the key is to increase

dietary zinc and calcium in the diet of high-risk children in Nigeria. How widespread clinical rickets is in many parts of the world remains a concern. (Free online.)

WHO Multicentre Growth Reference Study Group. 2006. *WHO Child Growth Standards: Length/Height-for-Age,   Weight-for-Age,   Weight-for-Length, Weight-for-Height and Body Mass Index-for-Age: Methods and Development.* Geneva, Switzerland: World Health Organization. http://www.who.int/childgrowth/standards/technical_report/en/. This is the reference document for the current globally accepted growth standards for infants and small children. (Free online.)

chapter five

Early school-age children (ages 4 to 8)

In identifying bone mineral needs of children in this age group, we have a new piece of science to consider. That is, beginning with children this age, some research studies have given supplements to children to determine the effect of calcium supplements on the rate at which bone is added to their skeleton.

One of the first pediatric calcium supplementation controlled trials was conducted in twins age 6 to 14 years of age (Johnston et al. 1992). Notably, the supplement showed a benefit of increased bone mineral only in those children who did not go through puberty during the three years of the trial. These data were interpreted as indicating that the optimal time for supplementation with calcium might be in younger, prepubertal children.

Studies since then have not really supported this concept of prepuberty being a key time for increasing bone mineral. Subsequent studies have, however, made it clear that calcium intake is important at a relatively young age, and it certainly is reasonable to consider tracking calcium intake in children in this age group.

In this age group, it becomes more common to consider the pros and cons of routine blood test screening for things such as dyslipidemias. Many health-care professionals consider testing for vitamin D status by measuring serum 25(OH)D during the routine pediatric examinations that children receive before starting school each year. Therefore, let us consider in this chapter if a healthy child needs to have their vitamin D status checked. This is an issue at any age, but is a good one to consider in this age group where it is a bit easier to draw a venous blood sample for serum 25(OH)D level than it is in younger children.

Should a healthy child have a routine or annual measurement of his serum vitamin D (25(OH)D) level?

A common question parents and medical caregivers have is whether an individual child should have their vitamin D status, as reflected by the serum 25(OH)D, measured. Sometimes this question is asked related to routine physical exams, and other times it is asked related to situations such as when a child falls, breaks a bone, and makes a Sunday afternoon visit to the local emergency room.

The IOM in its guidelines in 2011 did not specifically address this question (IOM 2011). That was not part of their mandate. They did, however, indicate that vitamin D insufficiency was uncommon in the United States. The Centers for Disease Control (CDC) has published information (Looker et al. 2011) that shows that levels that are very low for serum 25(OH)D (less than 12 ng/mL) occur in 1% to 2% of children under age 9, and 2% to 10% of children ages 9 to 18. In addition, levels that are between 12 and 20 ng/mL occur in approximately 10% of children less than 9 years of age, and 20% of children 9 to 18 years of age. More of the data from this report can be found in Chapters 6 and 7.

Overall, this means that the chance of having a low serum 25(OH)D, based on data in healthy American children is about 10% to 12% for children less than 9 years of age, and about 22% to 30% in children 9 to 18 years of age.

So, what are the pros and cons of getting a serum 25(OH)D level measured in a healthy child as a way of assessing vitamin D status?

Pros:

1. It is a straight-forward way of determining if a child is in the 10% to 30% of children and adolescents with genuinely low levels of serum 25(OH)D.
2. Results can be used to decide whether an individual child's current dietary intake of vitamin D is adequate to achieve a serum 25(OH)D level of at least 20 ng/mL, or if more vitamin D might be helpful in achieving this goal.

Cons:

1. The test to measure serum 25(OH)D requires a blood draw. It is currently not usually done from a fingerstick or a heelstick. This is not readily performed, especially in babies, in pediatric offices.
2. The test costs about $50 to $150 depending on the lab and test used. In healthy children, this may not be reimbursed by private insurance. Until there is strong evidence reviewed by truly independent groups that this testing has benefits to healthy children, we do not disagree with insurance refusal of reimbursement for healthy children. We all pay for such testing, even when the funding source is private insurance. This cost is in addition to any physician costs associated with obtaining the test if this is part of a physician visit.

3. The serum 25(OH)D test primarily measures exposure to vitamin D over the previous 6 weeks or so. Therefore, a test done in August will provide different results than one done in March. Although some people indicate this is a reason to do the testing, alternately, one could consider that this is a reason the test is not very useful for healthy children. To be absolutely certain of keeping a child's serum 25(OH)D level at a certain level every day would mandate checking the blood test several times a year. This would be a huge imposition on children and families as well as an intolerable cost for individuals and society. It would, however, make those who sell, conduct and analyze these tests, their consultants, and others very wealthy.

4. There are no data suggesting that healthy children benefit from routine monitoring of serum 25(OH)D levels or that intervention is needed beyond having a diet with or without supplements that contains the Recommended Dietary Allowance (RDA) of vitamin D. That is, no outcome studies in healthy children have shown that annual, or more frequent measuring of serum 25(OH)D level has a specific health benefit. This includes groups considered at high risk for deficient levels such as African Americans, Hispanics, and obese children.

5. Inevitably, doing one serum 25(OH)D test on any child will lead to recommendations to do more. In addition to the individual and societal costs, do we want to medicalize vitamin D requirements for children in this way? Would it not be better to just have children improve their diets or take supplements as needed? This description does not mean that there is no role for measuring serum 25(OH)D levels in children with chronic illnesses, other specialized needs, or health concerns.

On the whole, recognizing that the Preventative Task Force of the U.S. Public Health Service, the CDC, or the American Academy of Pediatrics (AAP) do not recommend routine serum 25(OH)D testing in healthy children, we see no reason for parents to ask for this test or for it to be performed in healthy children. Although this may be different in children with chronic illnesses, it is unlikely to be the case for a child with a typical fracture due to usual childhood activity. There is no evidence that usual activity-related fractures in children are connected to vitamin D levels or that being an active child constitutes a vitamin D–deficient disease. Nor is there any evidence that screening otherwise healthy children who have a single broken bone for their 25(OH)D level is the best way for us to spend our limited health care dollars.

Recently, the Endocrine Society, a scientific group which is not the same as the Pediatric Endocrine Society, (a group of pediatric endocrinologists), recommended that all African-American and Hispanic, as well as all obese children have their serum 25(OH)D measured (Holick et al. 2011). This subgroup of the population actually represents almost half of all children in the United States. The Endocrine Society provided no novel insight into this recommendation that was not available to the IOM and did not do any cost-benefit analysis. We strongly disagree with this recommendation. Healthy children, even those with dark skin, do not need to have blood tests drawn on a regular basis without a medical indication, and we do not need to fund these blood tests preferentially ahead of many other important public health needs until evidence suggests this is a truly useful way to spend a few billion of our health care dollars each year.

We are especially concerned about overtesting and overtreating children since about one-half of all children will have a blood test value for serum 25(OH)D in the 20 to 30 ng/mL range. We have already said that this value is not deficient or insufficient, based on both the best available science and public policy recommendations (IOM 2011). However, as we have noted, many laboratories report all serum 25(OH)D values less than 30 ng/mL or even 32 ng/mL, as *insufficient*, and well-meaning doctors or others will take action including high-dose supplements and repeated blood measurements. These are expensive over time and are done without any evidence of benefit in healthy children.

Therefore, what should be done? Sometimes one is evaluating a healthy child who has broken a bone during physical activity. First, if the child who has a fracture is one with a chronic illness or who has a special health-care or dietary situation, such as a vegan who avoids all dairy and does not take a calcium or vitamin D supplement, then it is certainly reasonable to test for bone health measures including a serum 25(OH)D level. Second, if the X-ray taken to look at the fracture seems to actually show severe bone demineralization or rickets, then, of course, a thorough evaluation should be done including a nutritional assessment and vitamin D testing which are among many tests that should be done. Finally, if an older infant has any clinical signs or history compatible with rickets, then this requires a full evaluation.

However, for most children, this just is not necessary. For the most part, children who are outside playing and break a bone have not done so because of a lack of vitamin D. Excluding situations we have listed above, the yield for this testing is low and the chance of excessive intervention may be high.

Bone density measurements and children

So far we have mostly talked about determining the need for nutrients such as calcium and vitamin D by describing how much calcium is absorbed and retained by the skeleton. Although useful and a key part of determining the Estimated Average Requirement (EAR) and RDA values, this method has severe limitations. These limitations include the technical challenges of determining absorption and the inability to accurately quantify some sources of nutrient losses such as sweat loss.

For bone health, there is a unique alternative approach involving the use of measurements of bone mineralization by a machine called a *Dual-Energy X-ray Absorptiometry* (DXA). In brief, this scan can measure the amount of bone in the body. It can either scan the entire body or just particular parts of the body such as the spine or hip for more specific measurements. The measurement of bone mineral includes both calcium and phosphorus and is called the *bone mineral content* (BMC). Based on this number, one can calculate fairly accurately, but not exactly, the total amount of calcium in the bone (Winzenberg and Jones 2011).

Although this is helpful, it is an approach that has lots of limitations. First, one has to decide which bones to measure and how to best measure them. DXA cannot measure the three-dimensional nature of bone. To account for this in adults, a correction of the total amount of bone mineral content (BMC) is made by estimating how much mineral there is in the three-dimensional space of real bones as opposed to the two-dimensional space measured by the DXA machine. This correction can be done in several ways, usually by dividing the BMC by the bone width or bone area, and calculating what is often called the *bone mineral density* (BMD). Although not a true density, BMD is a good approximation, and it is used widely in adult medicine for assessment of the spine and hip to determine risks of fracture.

In growing children, this calculation to determine BMD does not work as well as it does in adults due to the increase in bone area that occurs along with bone mineralization in this population group. Correcting BMC for bone size can be done in different ways, but these are imperfect. Furthermore, when we think about dietary mineral intake, we do not usually correct for body size or weight. For example, we do not think about a child who is 60 pounds needing half the amount of calcium in their diet as the same age child who weighs 120 pounds. For bone mineralization, we tend to also focus on the mineral *total*, the BMC, and not on the adjusted values such as the BMD (Van Kuijk 2010).

It gets even more confusing than this when we consider some newer techniques including those using ultrasound or computerized tomography (CT) scanners to measure bone, and the effects that growth of different parts of the body have on the whole body BMC. Nonetheless, for most purposes, in children, we tend to look at the whole amount of bone mineral, calculate the fraction of that which is calcium, and then determine the whole amount of calcium in the body.

Let us suppose that we measure the total body BMC on a child and it is about 855 grams (Figure 5.1). If we then remeasure the child exactly one year later, and he is 905 grams, then the child has gained 50 grams of bone mineral in 365 days or 50,000 mg/365 = 140 mg per day. Since BMC

DXA Results Summary:

Region	Area (cm²)	BMC (g)	BMD (g/cm²)	T - Score	PR (%)	Z - Score	AM (%)
L Arm	76.32	39.80	0.522				
R Arm	87.00	45.69	0.525				
L Ribs	75.93	35.72	0.470				
R Ribs	75.93	36.43	0.480				
T Spine	67.62	37.33	0.552				
L Spine	25.31	16.44	0.650				
Pelvis	100.84	80.07	0.794				
L Leg	164.51	127.05	0.772				
R Leg	156.21	121.72	0.779				
Subtotal	829.67	540.25	0.651				
Head	204.45	314.84	1.540				
Total	**1034.12**	**855.09**	**0.827**	**−3.9**	**69**	**0.4**	**103**

Total BMD CV 1.0%, ACF = 1.016, BCF = 0.948

Figure 5.1 A DXA scan showing the values for a 9-year-old child whose total body bone mineral is about 1000 grams. Note especially that the t-score is a –3.9 meaning that it is far below the mean for young adult normals. However, the appropriate reference here is the Z-score, the comparison with age and gender matched normal children, which is 0.4, slightly above average. (Figure courtesy of Roman Shypailo and Dr. Kenneth Ellis.)

is about 32.2% calcium, then the child gained 140 mg * 0.322 = about 50 mg of calcium each day (IOM 2011). This is somewhat below the average for this age, but is a value that might be of use in understanding what is happening to the child and his diet over time, especially if it is a child with a chronic illness. Note (Figure 5.1) the importance of using age and gender specific information to interpret the DXA scan. Using the standard of *adult young normal*, the 8-year-old boy in this example would have been profoundly deficient with a T-score (standard deviations below the young adult normal) of –3.9. Matched for age and gender, the child's bone mineralization was completely normal.

If we have a good idea of a child's average calcium intake during that period, then we can figure out how much they retained in their skeleton using the calculations provided above. More practically, we can determine the average amount of calcium that goes into the skeleton in a group of children of any given age. This value is called the rate of *calcium accretion* to the skeleton and it is used to determine how much calcium is needed in children to meet the usual amount that is accreted in the skeleton over any year.

Now then, in infants, we do not really use this information very much. But in toddlers and even more so in older children, we use this information to help us determine the target for how much calcium should go to the skeleton each year (calcium accretion). For 4- to 8-year-old children,

Table 5.1 How Many Children (Ages 4–13 Years Old)
Do Not Get Enough Calcium?

Life Stage Group	RDA (mg/day)	EAR (mg/day)	Mean Values of Estimated Intakes (mg/day)	% Below EAR
Males: 4–8 years old	1000	800	1059	21%
Males: 9–13 years old	1300	1100	1075	55%
Females: 4–8 years old	1000	800	951	35%
Females: 9–13 years old	1300	1100	967	68%

Source: NHANES 2005-2006, Calcium (mg/day): Percent of EAR Consumed in the United States from Food Sources Only Based on Mean Values of Estimated Intake.

the average amount of calcium that goes into the skeleton is about 120 to 140 mg per day, and it takes an average of 800 mg of calcium to reach that average (the EAR) and 1000 mg per day to assure that almost all children (97.5%) reach this amount (the RDA). In looking at usual dietary (not including supplement) intakes in 4- to 8-year-old children, the 50th percentile of calcium intake for boys is 1040 mg per day and for girls is 900 mg per day; therefore, about half of boys and about 60% to 65% of girls do not meet the RDA for calcium. Using the EAR cutoff method, and the EAR of 800 mg per day, then about 20% of boys and about 35% of girls do not meet the EAR intake for calcium (Tables 5.1 and 5.2). Note that supplement intake has a negligible effect on these numbers in this age group.

For vitamin D, the EAR remains 400 IU per day and the RDA 600 IU per day just as it is for toddlers 1 to 4 years old. Using dietary intake without supplements, 400 IU is at about the 90th percentile for boys and the 95th percentile for girls. The RDA of 600 IU per day is well above the 99th percentile of intakes for both boys and girls. This indicates that

Table 5.2 How Many Children (Ages 4–13 Years Old) Do Not Get Enough Calcium Even When Considering Intake from Supplements?

Life Stage Group	RDA (mg/day)	EAR (mg/day)	Mean Values of Estimated Intakes (mg/day)	% Below EAR
Males: 4–8 years old	1000	800	1087	19%
Males: 9–13 years old	1300	1100	1093	54%
Females: 4–8 years old	1000	800	974	32%
Females: 9–13 years old	1300	1100	988	65%

Source: Bailey RL, Dodd KW, Goldman JA, Gahche JJ, Dwyer JT, Moshfegh AJ, Sempos CT, and Picciano MF, 2010, Estimation of Total Usual Calcium and Vitamin D Intake in the United States, *Journal of Nutrition*, "Appendix H."

Table 5.3 How Many Children (Ages 4–13 Years Old)
Do Not Get Enough Vitamin D?

Life Stage Group	RDA (IU/day)	EAR (IU/day)	Mean Values of Estimated Intakes (IU/day)	% Below EAR
Males: 4–8 years old	600	400	256	89%
Males: 9–13 years old	600	400	224	92%
Females: 4–8 years old	600	400	216	96%
Females: 9–13 years old	600	400	208	93%

Source: NHANES 2005-2006, Vitamin D (IU/day): Percent of EAR Consumed in the United States from Food Sources Only Based on Mean Values of Estimated Intake.

Table 5.4 How Many Children (Ages 4–13 Years Old) Do Not Get Enough Vitamin D Even When Considering Intake from Supplements?

Life Stage Group	RDA (IU/day)	EAR (IU/day)	Mean Values of Estimated Intakes (IU/day)	% Below EAR
Males: 4–8 years old	600	400	372	63%
Males: 9–13 years old	600	400	300	80%
Females: 4–8 years old	600	400	316	76%
Females: 9–13 years old	600	400	308	77%

Source: Bailey RL, Dodd KW, Goldman JA, Gahche JJ, Dwyer JT, Moshfegh AJ, Sempos CT, and Picciano MF, 2010, Estimation of Total Usual Calcium and Vitamin D Intake in the United States, *Journal of Nutrition*, "Appendix H."

dietary sources alone are not meeting the needs of this age group. We will discuss more about dealing with this shortfall in children age 4 through adolescence (Tables 5.3 and 5.4) in the section on adolescents (Chapter 6).

How do you make sure a school-age child is getting enough vitamin D and calcium?

Giving a child 2 to 3 glasses of milk a day is often the best way to ensure a child is getting enough calcium and vitamin D. This, along with a few other sources of vitamin D and calcium, either naturally high in these nutrients or fortified with them, will help meet the goal. An 8-ounce cup of milk has 100 IU of vitamin D and about 300 mg of calcium (3 cups = 300 IU vitamin D and 900 mg calcium) (Figure 5.2).

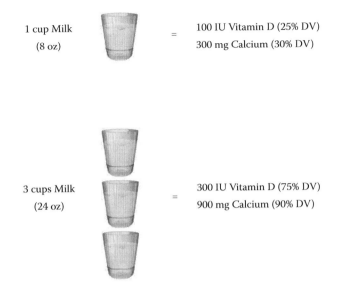

1 cup Milk   =   100 IU Vitamin D (25% DV)

(8 oz)   300 mg Calcium (30% DV)

3 cups Milk   =   300 IU Vitamin D (75% DV)

(24 oz)   900 mg Calcium (90% DV)

Figure 5.2 An 8-ounce cup of milk has 100 IU of vitamin D and about 300 mg of calcium (3 cups = 300 IU vitamin D and 900 mg calcium).

If a child does not like or cannot tolerate milk, there are other options. Lactose-intolerant children may still be able to drink milk infused with lactase, which has the same amount of vitamin D and calcium as other milk. Orange juice fortified with vitamin D and calcium (8 ounces has 100 IU of vitamin D and 350 mg of calcium) is widely available. It is important to specifically look at the label to see how much calcium or vitamin D is in the product.

Some cereals are fortified with extra vitamin D, but the market is easily split about 50/50 with cereals containing either 0 or 40 IU of vitamin D. For example, one serving of Raisin Nut Bran® by General Mills™ has 0 IU vitamin D, but Cheerios® by General Mills has 40 IU of vitamin D. And 1 cup of Total® cereal has 100 IU of vitamin D. At least that is all true today. Tomorrow, the numbers could change completely because we do not regulate these supplementation practices in these ranges in the United States. Margarine is the same story and can range from 0 to 80 IU of vitamin D per tablespoon of margarine. Yogurt covers the widest range. Some yogurts do not have any vitamin D while others have as much as 200 IU of vitamin D per serving. These product contents are constantly changing and one has to check the labels to be sure.

So it is easy to see that by just changing some of the brands in your grocery basket, you can easily increase the amount of vitamin D a child receives, without giving up taste. Some common foods and the wide variation of calcium and vitamin D intakes from them are shown in Table 5.5

Table 5.5 Calcium and Vitamin D Content of Yogurt

Brand of Yogurt (as of September 9, 2011)	Serving in Container	Calcium (mg/serv)	Vitamin D (IU/serv)
Dannon Activia® Light	6 oz	150	0
Brown Cow Farm® (all varieties)	8 oz	250	0
Dannon® Fruit on the Bottom	6 oz	250	0
Yoplait Kids® ("Calcium & vitamin D for strong bones")	3 oz	200	20
Dannon Dan-o-nino®	1.76 oz	200	24
Yoplait Gogurt®	2.25 oz	100	40
Yoplait Trix® yogurt ("Calcium & vitamin D for strong bones")	4 oz	100	40
Dannon Danimals Smoothie®	3.1 oz	250	40
Dannon Activia®	5.75 oz	150	60
Yoplait Greek®	6 oz	400	80
Stonyfield Greek®	6 oz	400	80
Stonyfield YoKids®	4 oz	200	100
Stonyfield Super Smoothie®	10 oz	400	100
Stonyfield Yo-baby®	4 oz	250	100
Lifeway ProBugs® cultured smoothie (gooberry pie)	5 oz	300	100
Stonyfield Yo-baby® Drinkable	6 oz	400	100
Yoplait Original®	6 oz	500	200

through Table 5.8. Recognize that these values are constantly changing but the table will give you an idea of the huge variation that is in the current marketplace.

Feeding children a healthy diet is an important, challenging, and worthy goal. By making simple changes to incorporate fortified foods and foods naturally rich in calcium and vitamin D, parents can easily keep familiar tastes that their children love while boosting their nutrition. Here is what we mean. Take a look at this *before* and *after* makeover of a typical 6-year-old child's daily menu (Tables 5.9 and 5.10). We just substituted different products and brands that are higher in calcium and vitamin D in order to reach the nutrient recommendations. You may even see places where this menu could be further improved to reach other recommendations for fruit and vegetable intake or whole grain intake. Our example is not meant to be an absolutely perfect day's menu but a way to demonstrate how you can be more deliberate about making food choices that improve calcium and vitamin D intakes.

Table 5.6 Calcium and Vitamin D Content of Cereal

Brand of Cereal (as of Sepember 9, 2011)	Serving Size	Calcium (mg/serv)	Vitamin D (IU/serv)
Special K® (original)	¾ c (30g)	0	0
General Mills Raisin Nut Bran®	¾ c (49g)	20	0
Kashi Go Lean®	¾ c (39g)	60	0
Quaker Life (original)®	¾ c (32g)	100	0
General Mills Fiber One®	½ c (30g)	100	0
Kellogg's Raisin Bran Crunch®	1 c (53g)	0	40
Special K® (vanilla almond)	¾ c (30g)	0	40
Post Raisin Bran®	1 c (59g)	20	40
Kellogg's Raisin Bran® (original)	1 c (59g)	20	40
Kellogg's Raisin Bran Extra®	1 c (49g)	20	40
General Mills Trix®	1 c (32g)	100	40
General Mills Lucky Charms®	¾ c (27g)	100	40
General Mills Cheerios® (all varieties)	¾ c (28g)	100	40
Total Whole Grain® (all Total varieties)	¾ c (30g)	1000	100

Table 5.7 Calcium and Vitamin D Content of Bread

Brand of Bread (as of September 9, 2011)	Calcium (mg/slice)	Vitamin D (IU/slice)
Nature's Own® 100% Whole Grain	0	0
Nature's Own® 100% Honey Wheat	0	0
Sara Lee Hearty & Delicious® 100% Whole Wheat	20	0
Mrs. Baird's® 100% Whole Wheat	20	0
Nature's Own® 100% Whole Wheat	40	0
Mrs. Baird's® White	40	0
Pepperidge Farm® 100% Whole Wheat	40	0
Orowheat® 100% Whole Wheat	60	0
WonderKids®	200	24
Sara Lee Soft & Smooth Plus® 100% Whole Wheat with Calcium & vitamin D	125	30
Sara Lee® White with calcium and vitamin D	125	30
Sara Lee Soft & Smooth Plus® Whole Grain White	125	30
Sara Lee® 100% Whole Wheat with calcium and vitamin D	125	30
Nature's Own® Whole Grain White	100	40

Table 5.8 Calcium and Vitamin D Content of Margarine

Brand of Margarine (as of September 9, 2011)	Calcium (mg/Tbsp)	Vitamin D (IU/Tbsp)
Land O' Lakes®	0	0
Brummel & Brown®	0	0
Benecol®	0	0
Promise Fat-Free®	0	0
Country Crock® spreadable butter and sticks	0	0
Country Crock® Honey Spread or Cinnamon Spread	100	0
Promise Buttery® Spread and Light Buttery Spread	0	60
Promise Active® Light Spread	0	60
Country Crock® Original, Light, and Churn Style	0	60
Country Crock® Calcium and Vitamin D	100	80

Picking a Multivitamin Supplement for Your School-Aged Child. What Should You Look For?

Whether all children need to take a daily multivitamin supplement is at best questionable. Nonetheless, these supplements do help provide key nutrients including calcium, vitamin D, iron, magnesium, and zinc that may be inadequate in the diets of many school children. Multivitamins should not, however, be expected to be the primary source for these nutrients, and there should be no reason to believe that good health mandates that all children take a multivitamin.

With all of that said, the question that many ask is, "Which multivitamin should I choose or recommend?" A quick trip to any grocery, pharmacy, health food store, or almost any store will find a shelf full of choices. Furthermore, they come as *brand names* or generics, and it can be a considerable task to figure out what is really in them or what to choose. The cost differences between generics and brand label may be large, leading to uncertainty as to whether there is a quality difference between these products.

We have already noted that foods cannot list the actual amounts of the micronutrients in them. This is not true of supplements, however. They are regulated separately and can, and do, tell you what is in them, and what form the micronutrient is in. Sometimes they come, stated on the bottle or on the Internet, with claims of superior bioavailability (the proportion absorbed and used by the body).

Table 5.9 Typical *Before* Menu in a Sample Before and After Menu Makeover for a 6-Year-Old Child

Meal	Calcium (mg)	Vitamin D (IU)
Breakfast:		
1 biscuit	38	7
1 tbsp jam	0	0
1 banana	0	0
4 fl oz orange juice	0	0
Lunch:		
2 slices bread	0	0
2-3 oz deli turkey meat	0	0
1 slice provolone cheese	212	6
1 snack bag chips	0	0
6 fl oz water	0	0
Afternoon Snack:		
1 oz bag potato chips	8	0
1 pouch Capri-Sun®	6	0
Dinner:		
½ cup spaghetti noodles	5	0
½ cup spaghetti sauce with meat	34	0
1 small slice garlic bread	15	3
6 fl oz skim milk	225	86
1 small brownie	14	8
TOTAL	557 mg/day	113 IU/day

There is no perfect way to sort this out, but here are some helpful ideas:

1. First, look at the front of the bottle. If it says "For Women", then they generally mean that it is designed for adolescent girls or adult women who are regularly having menstrual periods and need supplemental iron if they do not regularly eat a lot of iron fortified foods or red meat. If it says "For Men" then generally they have little or any iron in them as adult men do not commonly need extra iron and may be harmed by it. If it says "For Over 50 Years," it will usually have little or no iron due to lower iron requirements for this age group.

Table 5.10 *After* Menu in a Sample Before and After Menu Makeover for a
6-Year-Old Child

Meal	Calcium (mg)	Vitamin D (IU)
Breakfast:		
¾ cup Cheerios	100	40
½ cup skim milk	150	50
1 banana	0	0
4 fl oz calcium & vitamin D-fortified orange juice	150	50
Lunch:		
2 slices whole grain white bread	300	100
2–3 oz deli turkey meat	50	0
1 slice provolone cheese	212	6
1 snack bag chips	0	0
8 fl oz chocolate skim milk	300	100
Afternoon Snack:		
6 oz Yoplait Original Yogurt	500	200
1 pouch Capri-Sun	6	0
Dinner:		
½ cup spaghetti noodles	5	0
½ cup spaghetti sauce with meat	34	3
1 small slice garlic bread	15	3
8 fl oz skim milk	300	100
1 small brownie	14	0
TOTAL	2136 mg/day	660 IU/day

2. Next look and see if the vitamin is *broad* in its contents. There typically should be more than a dozen vitamins (not all named as vitamins) including vitamin A, C, D, and E, and a range of minerals including calcium, magnesium, zinc, and copper. Any supplement used for adolescent or young adult females should have folic acid in it. Supplements designed for the elderly usually have vitamin B_{12} included as well.

3. Next, look at the amounts in the supplements. Most supplements will provide 100% of the Daily Value for most nutrients, and that is what you should look for. However, this is not going to be true of all nutrients. For example, the Daily Value for calcium is 1000 mg each

day. Taking a pill or multiple pills with large amounts of calcium is unlikely to be helpful because that much calcium cannot be absorbed by the body at one time, and may cause side effects including constipation. Instead, a good multivitamin supplement should only have 200 to 500 mg of calcium.

4. There should be few if any nutrients in which the % Daily Value is above 100%. Supplements are not generally designed to be the only way in which individuals receive all of their vitamins and minerals. An exception here sometimes is vitamin D, in which some supplements designed for adults now contain over 400 IU even in multivitamin pills. Multivitamin supplements containing 1000 IU are common and safe in a multivitamin for adults and older children since the upper level for total intake in adolescents and adults is 4000 IU per day.

5. Additionally, look at the chemical form in which key minerals are found. This can be especially important for vitamin D, in which it is usually best to choose vitamin D_3 (cholecalciferol) as opposed to vitamin D_2 (ergocalciferol). It can also be important for iron. Some supplements will contain iron in the chemical form bound to amino acids. These may be better tolerated and more readily absorbed by some people. In general, however, for routine multivitamins, the common forms of ferrous sulfate or ferrous fumarate are well tolerated because the amount of iron is not very high. Those individuals who get an upset stomach related to iron should try the specialized forms. These are more expensive but may be the only forms that some individuals can tolerate.

6. Finally, look to see if there are other nutrients that might be beneficial in the supplement, such as omega-3 fatty acids. These are gaining in popularity in most multivitamins; however, the evidence of their benefit in small children is not compelling at present. Still, overall health benefits are likely real, and it is worthwhile to consider including these especially for children with limited fish intake.

Consider using reliable online references such as *Consumer Reports* to check out individual brands. Discuss options with pharmacists or others who have experience with individual supplement brands.

References

Holick MF, Binkley NC, Bischoff-Ferrari HA, Gordon CM, Hanley DA, Heaney RP, Murad MH, and Weaver CM. 2011. Evaluation, treatment, and prevention of vitamin D deficiency: An endocrine society clinical practice guideline. *J Clin Endocrinol Metab* 96:1911–30. See annotation in Chapter 2 "References." (Not free online.)

Institute of Medicine. 2011. *Dietary Reference Intakes for Calcium and vitamin D.* Washington, DC: National Academy Press. See annotation in Chapter 2 "References."

Johnston CC, Miller JZ, Slemenda CW, Reister TK, Hui S, Christian JC, and Peacock M. 1992. Calcium supplementation and increases in bone mineral density in children. *N Engl J Med* 327:82–7. One of the first controlled trials of calcium supplementation in children showed a benefit for those who were prepubertal but not those who were pubertal during the study. Whether these benefits persisted was not reported in this manuscript. This is one of the classic studies that had a profound affect on future calcium-related research and the view of the nutrition community on calcium supplementation in children. (Free online.)

Looker AC, Johnson CL, Lacher DA, Pfeiffer CM, Schleicher RL, and Sempos CT. 2011. Vitamin D status: United States, 2001–2006. *NCHS Data Brief.* March (59):18. http://www.cdc.gov/nchs/data/databriefs/db59.htm. A very clear representation of the status of vitamin D in the United States based on serum 25-OHD levels from the CDC. (Free online.)

Van Kuijk C. 2010. Pediatric bone densitometry. *Radiol Clin North Am* 48:623–7. This is a review of pediatric specific issues related to DXA use. DXA is a very safe modality for determining body composition and bone mineral status. It should commonly be used for children with almost all chronic illnesses. It is crucial, however, that the scan be interpreted by someone familiar with pediatric values. The reference ranges used in adults are not age and gender appropriate for children and this can be confusing to those not familiar with pediatric standards. (Not free online.)

Winzenberg T and Jones G. 2011. Dual-energy X-ray absorptiometry. *Aust Fam Physician* 40:43–4. This is brief summary of DXA issues that can be helpful to those not able to access other fee-based online articles. (Free online.)

chapter six

Adolescents

What happens to bone and when does it happen?

We typically think of adolescence as being synonymous with *teenage* and ascribe an age of 13 to 19 years for this time period. However, bones, especially those of girls, are operating on a different *clock*. During the adolescent growth spurt, over a period of about 5 to 6 years, the body will gain about two-thirds of all of its bone minerals. By the end of adolescence, an individual will have about 95% of their maximum bone mineral, with the potential for adding a small amount later on.

We now have a number of Dual-Energy X-ray Absorptiometry (DXA) studies and other research to demonstrate that this incredible increase in bone mineral begins earlier than we might expect and ends sooner than we might like. It is driven largely by the earliest release of pubertal hormones and ends when the hormonal changes of puberty end. It is different in boys and in girls, and it has a huge age range of occurrence, just as puberty does.

With that said, typically, the beginnings of the pubertal bone mineral growth spurt occur as early as about age 9 to 10 years in girls and 10 to 12 years in boys. In girls, it has nearly ended by around age 14 to 16. In boys, the end is often later, up to 18 to 20 years of age (Abrams 2003). A small amount of increase continues after that time, but very little bone mineral is added after the end of the pubertal growth spurt (Baxter-Jones et al. 2011). A fascinating but not well-explained recent study even suggests that vitamin D status may be related to the timing of puberty. That is, girls in the South American nation of Colombia with serum 25(OH)D values less than 20 ng/mL had their first menstrual period (menarche) at an average age of 11.8 years compared with those whose serum 25(OH)D value was greater than 30 ng/mL who reached menarche at an average age of 12.6 years (Villamor et al. 2011). Much more information is needed to confirm and explain this finding, however, and there is no suggestion that premature puberty is related to serum 25(OH)D levels, especially if greater than 20 ng/mL.

What does this early onset of bone growth and mineralization mean? It means that fighting with your 16-year-old daughter about a healthy diet rich in calcium and vitamin D–containing foods is basically fighting a battle that is nearly over in its most important form. The increase in calcium requirement due to more rapid bone growth begins well before the teenage years. This is the time when more dietary calcium is needed and the time to ensure adequate vitamin D and other nutrient intake. It is important to continue a good bone healthy diet later in adolescence, but the time to focus on this begins at age 9 to 10, not age 15 or 16 (Abrams, O'Brien, and Stuff 1996).

What drives bone mineralization during puberty and what is meant by peak bone mass?

There is still a lot to be learned about how and why bones increase in size and mineralization so rapidly in such a short time during puberty. It appears that there is a marked increase in calcium absorption from the diet during puberty that is largely based on changes in pubertal hormones, including estrogen and growth hormone.

One might think that greatly increasing the serum level of vitamin D, 25(OH)D, would be important in order to increase the amount of calcium absorbed by the body. Interestingly, several recent and detailed studies suggest that this is not the case. It is clear that having *enough* vitamin D is needed, but it is also fairly clear that having a certain serum level of 25(OH)D above 15 to 20 ng/mL does not increase calcium absorption or bone formation in adolescents. That is, there is no reason based on currently available science to mandate a minimum serum 25(OH)D of 30 ng/mL or more to optimize calcium absorption or bone mineralization (Abrams et al. 2005; Park et al. 2010; Abrams, Hicks, and Hawthorne 2009).

In reviewing this information, the Institute of Medicine (IOM) (2011) established an *average* level of 25(OH)D in the serum, an Estimated Average Requirement (EAR) level of 16 ng/mL, and a Recommended Dietary Allowance (RDA) level of 20 ng/mL. These values were set for all age groups over 1 year of age, recognizing that there was not good information for setting these values in the first year of life. This recommendation was virtually identical to that from the Pediatric Endocrine Society (Misra et al. 2008). We know based on national survey data that about 7% of male adolescents and 10% of female adolescents are at risk for vitamin D *deficiency*, defined as a serum 25(OH)D below 12 ng/mL, and that about 22% of males and 24% of females are at risk for vitamin D *inadequacy* defined as a serum 25(OH)D below 20 ng/mL (Figures 6.1 and 6.2).

Peak bone mass is the maximum total body Bone Mineral Content (BMC) that a person achieves. The importance of the peak bone mass is that once bone loss begins, it tends to be lost at a relatively fixed rate. Therefore, the higher one starts and the greater the peak bone mass, the

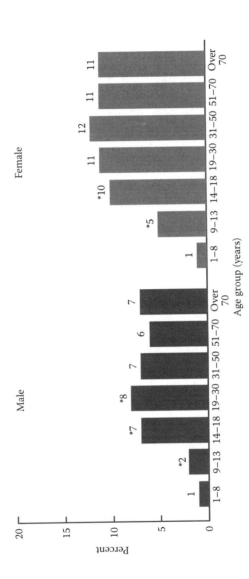

Figure 6.1 Prevalence at risk of vitamin D deficiency (CDC). This graph shows that 2-7% of boys and 5-10% of girls ages 9 to 18 have very low 25(OH)D levels below 30 nmol/L (equivalent to 12 ng/mL). Still, this is not a trivial amount of the population. (Looker AC, Johnson CL, Lacher DA, Pfeiffer CM, Schleicher RL, Sempos CT, Vitamin D Status: United States, 2001–2006, NCHS Data Brief, 2011, March (59):1–8.)

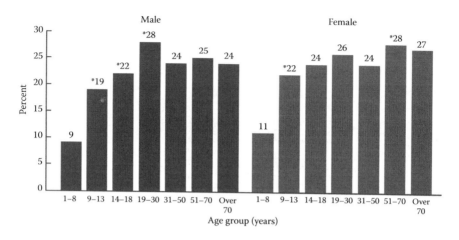

Figure 6.2 Prevalence at risk of inadequacy (CDC). This growth shows that 19-22% of boys and 22-24% of girls have 25(OH)D levels between 30 and 49 nmol/L (about 12 to 20 ng/mL). Although defined as insufficient, the clinical consequences of 25(OH)D levels in this range is less certain. (Looker AC, Johnson CL, Lacher DA, Pfeiffer CM, Schleicher RL, Sempos CT, Vitamin D Status: United States, 2001–2006, NCHS Data Brief, 2011, March (59):1–8.)

longer it takes until bone loss reaches a point at which fractures are more likely to occur due to trauma such as falling.

As we noted before, most girls reach nearly this level at about age 16 and boys at about age 18. A very small increase, usually about 5%, can occur in the late teenage years and in the early twenties, with the absolute final peak in bone mineralization usually occurring between ages 25 and 30. After that, BMC stays fairly constant for 10 to 15 years and then begins to decline, most rapidly around the time of menopause in women but also in men in their 50s and 60s.

There is little doubt that the most important determinant of peak bone mass for anyone is his or her genetic makeup. We are all born having multiple genes which affect our peak bone mass. Although scientists debate exactly how much of the variation in peak bone mass is due to genetics and how much is due to environmental factors including diet, a reasonable estimate is that at least 80% of the variability between individuals in bone mineralization and bone mass is genetic. We cannot change our gender, race, or vitamin D–related genes, but we can affect that other 20%, and this can be a big difference. Even an increase in bone mineral of 3% to 5% can have a large impact on the risk of fracturing a bone in later life.

Amount and source of calcium and vitamin D in adolescent diets

Knowing that dairy sources make up the largest source of calcium in the diet and that many adolescents slow down or stop drinking milk in favor of sodas, or sports and energy drinks, it should come as no surprise that adolescents have low calcium and vitamin D intakes overall.

Most of the discussion about calcium and vitamin D intake in smaller children also applies to adolescents. However, there are a couple of key differences. The most important of these is that the RDA for calcium for ages 9 to 18 goes up to 1300 mg per day, an amount well above the usual intake of this age group. The difference is particularly large for adolescent girls. Very few girls have an intake this high. Remembering our discussion that 1300 mg per day is only an approximation of the real need, the question becomes, what is the minimum needed and what should be done when calcium intakes from the diet do not reach that minimum?

As far as a minimum amount, research generally suggests that the *least* amount of calcium an adolescent should have is about 800 to 1100 mg per day. This is not the *optimal* amount to maximize bone mineralization, but it is an amount that appears to at least come reasonably close to meeting bone growth needs. The IOM set 1100 mg per day as the EAR. At intakes below about 600 mg per day, on a typical American diet, a fairly large deficiency in total calcium absorbed by the body exists (Abrams et al. 2004).

Getting calcium intakes into the 1100 mg per day and above range is a real challenge not met by many adolescents, especially girls (Table 6.1). If an individual's dietary calcium intakes are consistently below 1100 mg per day despite best efforts at providing dairy and fortified foods, then we would recommend consideration of a calcium supplement, especially one in the form of a multivitamin with minerals (Table 6.2). The calcium in the supplement would typically be 200 to 500 mg, and there should be 400 IU of vitamin D in each supplement pill. Other nutrients, including magnesium, iron, and zinc should also be present. A multivitamin that contains calcium in the form of calcium carbonate is fine for this age group when a supplement is used.

Table 6.1 How Many Teenagers Do Not Get Enough Calcium?

Life Stage Group	RDA (mg/day)	EAR (mg/day)	Mean Values of Estimated Intakes (mg/day)	% Below EAR
Males: 14–18 years old	1300	1100	1270	44%
Females: 14–18 years old	1300	1100	876	78%

Source: NHANES 2005–2006, Calcium (mg/day): Percent of EAR Consumed in the United States from Food Sources Only Based on Mean Values of Estimated Intake.

Table 6.2 How Many Teenagers Do Not Get Enough Calcium Even When Considering Intake from Supplements?

Life Stage Group	RDA (mg/day)	EAR (mg/day)	Mean Values of Estimated Intakes (mg/day)	% Below EAR
Males: 14–18 years old	1300	1100	1297	41%
Females: 14–18 years old	1300	1100	918	75%

Source: Bailey RL, Dodd KW, Goldman JA, Gahche JJ, Dwyer JT, Moshfegh AJ, Sempos CT, and Picciano MF, 2010, Estimation of Total Usual Calcium and Vitamin D Intake in the United States, *Journal of Nutrition*, "Appendix H."

Table 6.3 How Many Teenagers Do Not Get Enough Vitamin D?

Life Stage Group	RDA (IU/day)	EAR (IU/day)	Mean Values of Estimated Intakes (IU/day)	% Below EAR
Males: 14–18 years old	600	400	240	80%
Females: 14–18 years old	600	400	148	96%

Source: NHANES 2005–2006, Vitamin D (IU/day): Percent of EAR Consumed in the United States from Food Sources Only Based on Mean Values of Estimated Intake.

However, if a child or adolescent complains about side effects from calcium carbonate such as constipation, it is reasonable to try calcium citrate or another form of calcium. Usually, this should not be necessary. Parents should avoid having children take such high amounts of calcium from supplements. Currently, even those children who avoid milk completely have many other alternatives for obtaining 600 to 800 mg each day of calcium from their diet, so that very high-dose supplements are not needed to reach either the EAR or the RDA levels of intake.

Teenagers often do not get enough vitamin D either (Tables 6.3 and 6.4). The new EAR for adolescents 14 to 18 years of age is 400 IU per day

Table 6.4 How Many Teenagers Do Not Get Enough Vitamin D Even When Considering Intake from Supplements?

Life Stage Group	RDA (IU/day)	EAR (IU/day)	Mean Values of Estimated Intakes (IU/day)	% Below EAR
Males: 14–18 years old	600	400	276	77%
Females: 14–18 years old	600	400	200	84%

Source: Bailey RL, Dodd KW, Goldman JA, Gahche JJ, Dwyer JT, Moshfegh AJ, Sempos CT, and Picciano MF, 2010, Estimation of Total Usual Calcium and Vitamin D Intake in the United States, *Journal of Nutrition*, "Appendix H."

Table 6.5 Typical *Before* Menu in a Sample Before and After
Menu for 14-Year-Old Girl

Meal	Calcium (mg)	Vitamin D (IU)
Breakfast:		
1 Quaker Chewy® granola bar	5	0
Lunch:		
2 slices Mrs. Baird's white bread	76	0
3 oz deli turkey	8	3
1 oz bag potato chips	8	0
1 banana	5	0
1 pudding cup	58	0
12 fl oz soda	7	0
Afternoon Snack:		
½ bag microwave popcorn	3	0
1 pouch Capri-Sun	6	0
Dinner:		
2 slices pepperoni pizza	335	17
20 fl oz soda	12	0
1 brownie	14	8
TOTAL	527 mg/day	28 IU/day

of vitamin D; however, most teens fall far short of that with 80% of males below the EAR and 96% of females below the EAR.

Helping adolescents to make wise food choices is critical to a healthy diet. By emphasizing foods and beverages that are rich in calcium and vitamin D, as well as fortified products, intakes can be maximized to reach recommended levels in many children. Take a look at these sample menus to see what we mean (Tables 6.5 and 6.6). We do not intend for these menus to display the absolute healthiest diet possible. For example, they clearly do not meet all the concerns of the Dietary Guidelines for Americans (www.dietaryguidelines.gov). However, from the point of view of calcium and vitamin D intake, one can see that by switching a few foods and making simple changes, one can greatly increase calcium and vitamin D levels in the diet.

It might be helpful to know that when adolescents do include milk in their diet, 55% of the time it is as plain white milk as a beverage (Figure 6.3).

Table 6.6 *After* Menu in a Sample Before and After Menu for a 14-Year-Old Girl

Meal	Calcium (mg)	Vitamin D (IU)
Breakfast:		
1 Nutri-Grain® granola bar	200	0
8 fl oz calcium & vitamin D-fortified orange juice	300	100
Lunch:		
2 slices Mrs. Baird's® whole grain white bread	400	80
3 oz deli turkey	8	3
1 oz bag potato chips	8	0
1 banana	5	0
1 pudding cup	58	0
8 fl oz skim milk	300	100
Afternoon Snack:		
½ bag microwave popcorn	3	0
8 fl oz skim milk	300	100
Dinner:		
2 slices pepperoni pizza	335	17
20 fl oz soda	12	0
1 brownie	14	8
After Dinner:		
6 oz Yoplait® Original Yogurt	500	200
TOTAL	2443 mg/day	608 IU/day

The role of exercise in bone health

Those who care for children are increasingly challenged to provide enough physical activity for them. There is little doubt that one of the causes of the obesity epidemic in children is not enough physical activity. It is important to understand the basic role exercise has in bone health. First, it is unquestionable that exercise has a strong positive effect on bone growth in children. There is even some evidence that this is true in premature infants, although caution needs to be used in this group. Exercise does not directly increase calcium deposition in bone, but it does enlarge and strengthen growing bones and the muscles that support them. There is reasonably strong evidence that, for growing bones, exercise is at least as important as maintaining a high-calcium intake, and it might be more important.

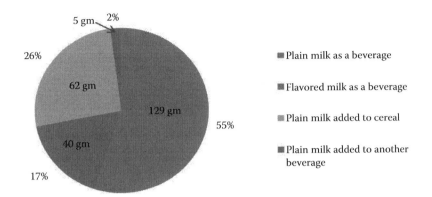

Figure 6.3 Milk intake in adolescents. Perhaps surprisingly, the majority of intake is from unflavored milk.

Specker and coworkers (Specker and Vukovich 2007) have studied the interaction of nutrition and exercise in bone mineral growth and development in childhood. They demonstrated the importance of exercise in a variety of groups of children in enhancing bone health. Several years ago, in reviewing this area, they concluded "Current evidence suggests that regular weight-bearing exercise and adequate dietary calcium intakes (around 1000 mg per day) may be required to optimize bone health; however, exercise would appear to be more important for optimizing bone strength because it has a direct effect (e.g., via loading) on bone mass and structural properties, whereas nutritional factors appear to have an indirect effect (e.g., via hormonal factors) on bone mass."

However, some caution must also be noted on the other side of this discussion. Excessive exercise combined with inadequate nutrient intake is the basis for what is called the *female athletic triad.* Although this designation is controversial, in general, the triad consists of an eating disorder, decreased or absent menstrual periods, and osteoporosis. This disorder is increasingly being diagnosed in young athletes and provides some caution to the role of exercise in health, including bone health (Nattiv et al. 2007).

What Can Children Learn about Food Labels to Help with Better Nutrition?

Children, especially teenagers and preteens (ages 9 to 12) can be taught to read and understand food labels (Figure 6.4). The first thing is to show them where to locate the Serving Size and Servings per Container. Teach children that one package does not necessarily mean one serving. Consider that sinfully delicious pint of ice cream in your freezer. The Serving Size on that

Nutrition Facts

Serving Size 1/2 cup (88g)
Servings Per Container 4

Amount Per Serving

Calories 180   Calories from Fat 70

                                                    %Daily Value*

Total Fat 8g	**12%**
Saturated Fat 6g	**30%**
Trans Fat 0g	
Cholesterol 35mg	**12%**
Sodium 75mg	**3%**
Total Carbohydrate 21g	**7%**
Dietary Fiber 0g	**0%**
Sugars 21g	
Protein 5g	

Vitamin A 6%	•	Vitamin C 2%
Calcium 15%	•	Iron 0%

* Percent Daily Values are based on a 2,000 calorie diet. Your Daily Values may be higher or lower depending on your calorie needs:

	Calories:	2,000	2,500
Total Fat	Less than	65g	80g
Sat Fat	Less than	20g	25g
Cholesterol	Less than	300mg	300mg
Sodium	Less than	2,400mg	2,400mg
Total Carb		300g	375g
Dietary Fiber		25g	30g

Figure 6.4 Sample food label for ice cream.

yummy treat says one-half cup per serving and that there are 4 servings in that pint.

Next, put a child's math skills to practical use and teach them that if they were to eat 1 serving of the ice cream, they would get the amount of nutrients listed on the food label. This idea is somewhat flawed, however, since they may not need 2000 calories per day or have the same need as the Daily Value. If they eat the whole container, which is 4 servings, then they should multiply all the nutrients by 4 to find out how much nutrition they are really getting. The next step is a little harder and might be too hard for the younger children in this group to understand. What if you decide to eat three-quarters of a cup of ice cream? Or what if you decide to eat about one and one-quarter cups? It becomes a little harder to do the math in order to figure out exactly what you are eating, but the idea is the same. If you eat more than the amount stated in the serving size, you have to recognize that all the nutrients on the food label will increase.

Then, it is time to talk about nutrients. At this age, children already know that some things are good for them and other things are bad for them. It is more important to emphasize overall healthiness in a diet rather than to focus too much on naming a single nutrient. But you can talk with a child about how their bodies need less of things like fat, saturated fat, cholesterol, sodium, and sugars. Growing bodies need more vitamins (such as vitamins A and C), and minerals (such as iron and calcium). (These are the only four vitamins and minerals required by law to be on the food label unless the manufacturer makes a claim about another nutrient). This is a concept a child can understand. Further discussions from here can also go into what these nutrients do in your body and why they are healthy or not as healthy, as well as balance and moderation.

A good use of the Daily Value is to know if a food is generally low or high in a particular nutrient. Low is not always bad and high is not always good. That is why it is important to teach children which nutrients we need more of and which ones we need less of. A good rule of thumb is the *5 and 20 Rule*. A nutrient's Daily Value is low if it is 5% or less. If the nutrient you are looking at on the Food Label is low in saturated fat, then that is a good thing and a healthy choice. If it is low in calcium or another nutrient we may need more of, then low is not such a good choice. If the nutrient's Daily Value is 20% or more, then that is considered high. Again, if the food you are evaluating has more than 20% of the Daily Value for sodium, you might want to consider another choice. If the food has more than 20% of the Daily Value for vitamin C, it may be a good choice.

One food is not the equivalent of just one single nutrient. Just because a food is high in one healthy nutrient does not mean that it is the best food overall for your child to eat. Combination foods are particularly complex: frozen organic pizza may be high in vitamin C because of the tomato sauce and high in calcium because of the cheese, but it could also be high in sodium, fat, and calories, depending on the brand and other toppings.

With these tips, and more like it produced by the Food and Drug Administration's (FDA) *Spot the Block* food label educational campaign, children can learn to interpret low and high values of healthy and less healthy nutrients and make the food label work for them (http://www.cartoonnetwork.com/promos/201004_fda/index.html). Good news! These tips work to help adults figure out the food label too.

Energy Drinks and Children

In June 2011, the American Academy of Pediatrics (AAP) released a recommendation that strongly encouraged tightly limiting children's access to both *energy drinks* and *sports drinks* (Committee on Nutrition and the Council on Sports Medicine and Fitness 2011). This report may have surprised many parents and healthcare providers, who thought that these were good alternatives to soda. Therefore, we would like to discuss the rationale behind the recommendation including how it relates to bone health.

First, children, like anyone else, typically have a certain amount of fluids they drink each day. In recommending what those fluids should consist of, important considerations include energy (calories), providing nutrients needed for growth (e.g., calcium and vitamin D), and avoiding fluids that children do not need (e.g., caffeine).

On the whole, the two best drinks that meet these requirements by providing both fluids and nutrients are water and milk. As we have noted, children should get at least 2 to 3 servings of milk each day. The rest of the fluids are best provided by water. The price is right, the calorie content is perfect for most children, and the physiology is ideal! Water and milk are a great source of most fluid intake. Water does not need added minerals, vitamins, or even sugar. It does not need to come from a well across the world or cost a dollar a bottle either ($5 at baseball games).

Now, for children who are exercising in a serious fashion, some sports drink intake is acceptable and can help them replenish their electrolytes. However, many children do not use them this way. Instead they use them as a *water replacement* throughout the day. Sports drinks and energy drinks have substantial calories and in some cases unneeded extras like caffeine.

In general, we are not fans of an absolute approach to nutrition. An occasional nonalcoholic illicit beverage, such as a soda, or a sports or energy drink, will hardly ruin a child's health. But, that does not mean that parents should buy them for routine home consumption or that schools should be promoting these in the cafeteria or vending machines. Sports drinks are not *better* than sodas as a water replacement. The AAP has this correct, and parents along with those who advise them should consider carefully when choosing how to fill up the refrigerator.

References

Abrams SA. 2003. Normal acquisition and loss of bone mass. *Horm Res* 60(Suppl 3):71–6. This is a review of the natural pattern of bone mineral acquisition and loss over the lifespan. (Not free online.)

Abrams SA, Griffin IJ, Hawthorne KM, Gunn SK, Gundberg CM, and Carpenter TO. 2005. Relationships among vitamin D levels, parathyroid hormone, and calcium absorption in young adolescents. *J Clin Endocrinol Metab* 90:5576–81. This is our research study showing that in children whose serum 25(OH)D level is above about 12 ng/mL, there is little relationship between serum 25(OH)D and calcium absorption. (Free online.)

Abrams SA, Griffin IJ, Hicks PD, and Gunn SK. 2004. Pubertal girls only partially adapt to low dietary calcium intakes. *J Bone Min Res* 19:759–763. We put girls on a very low calcium diet. They adapted partially by increasing their calcium absorption efficiency. However, this was not even close to enough to keep them from retaining the same amount of calcium they would have received had they been on a normal calcium diet. (Free online.)

Abrams SA, Hicks PD, and Hawthorne KM. 2009. Higher serum 25–hydroxyvitamin D levels in school-age children are inconsistently associated with increased calcium absorption. *J Clin Endocrinol Metab* 94:2421–7. This is complicated. There is a very tiny effect of vitamin D levels on calcium absorption but overall, at serum 25(OH)D values over about 15 ng/mL, the effect is minimal. (Free online.)

Abrams SA, O'Brien KO, and Stuff JE. 1996. Changes in calcium kinetics associated with menarche. *J Clin Endocrinol Metab* 81:2017–2020. When it comes to bones, it all happens well before the teenage years. Begin to focus on a bone healthy diet with 9- and 10-year-old children. Do not wait until age 13. (Free online.)

Baxter-Jones AD, Faulkner RA, Forwood MR, Mirwald RL, and Bailey DA. 2011. Bone mineral accrual from 8 to 30 years of age: An estimation of peak bone mass. *J Bone Miner Res* 26:1729–39. This is a very recent article confirming that the pubertal growth spurt is when it mostly all happens in terms of bone mineral accrual. By the early 20s it is virtually all over for increasing peak bone mass. (Not free online.)

Committee on Nutrition and the Council on Sports Medicine and Fitness. 2001. Sports drinks and energy drinks for children and adolescents: Are they appropriate? *Pediatrics* 127:1182–1189. The AAP does not think so. Children should mostly drink water or milk, that is, reasonably affordable water without vitamins that will mostly get flushed away in the urine. (Free online.)

Institute of Medicine. 2011. *Dietary Reference Intakes for Calcium and vitamin D.* Washington, DC: National Academy Press. See annotation in Chapter 2 "References."

Misra M, Pacaud D, Petryk A, Collett-Solberg PF, Kappy M, and Drug and Therapeutics Committee of the Lawson Wilkins Pediatric Endocrine Society. 2008. Vitamin D deficiency in children and its management: Review of current knowledge and recommendations. *Pediatrics* 122:398–417. Not to be confused with the *Endocrine Society* that had very different recommendations. We trust the pediatric endocrine group, which is related to children and recommend using this article as a guide. (Free online.)

Nattiv A, Loucks AB, Manore MM, Sanborn CF, Sundgot-Borgen J, Warren MP and American College of Sports Medicine (ACSM). 2007. American College of Sports Medicine position stand: The female athlete triad. *Med Sci Sports Exerc* 39:1867–82. This is the official sports medicine statement about the female athlete triad and explores why it is a position *stand* instead of a position *statement*. (Not free online.)

Park CY, Hill KM, Elble AE, Martin BR, DiMeglio LA, Peacock M, McCabe GP, and Weaver CM. 2010. Daily supplementation with 25 μg cholecalciferol does not increase calcium absorption or skeletal retention in adolescent girls with low serum 25 hydroxyvitamin. *D. J Nutr* 140:2139–44. This is more information that vitamin D levels and supplementation do not drive calcium absorption in adolescents except when the serum 25(OH) is very low. (Free online at the end of 2011.)

Specker B and Vukovich M. 2007. Evidence for an interaction between exercise and nutrition for improved bone health during growth. *Med Sport Sci* 51:50–63. It is a good idea for growing children and adolescents to build strong bones with exercise, while maintaining an adequate calcium intake. Makes sense to us. (Not free online.)

Villamor E, Maric C, Mora-Plazas M, and Baylin A. 2011. Vitamin D deficiency and age at menarche: A prospective study. *Am J Coin Nutr.* 94:1020–5. This is a fascinating but not well-explained study from Colombia suggesting a link between age at puberty and vitamin D deficiency. This is a challenging link to make, and there may well be unidentified covariates controlling this relationship rather than a real effect of vitamin D. Still, this is an area for future investigation. It should not be overinterpreted though as saying that premature pubertal development is due to inadequate vitamin D status. (Not free online until late 2012.)

chapter seven

Pregnancy and lactation

Fetal bone mineralization

Beginning around the middle of the second trimester, the fetus requires about 200 to 300 mg of calcium every day to mineralize its bones. This might not seem like a lot for an adult woman to provide her fetus, but it is! Young adults are generally in calcium *balance*. That means that they are neither gaining nor losing calcium from their skeleton. Typically, that means that a young adult nonpregnant woman who has 1000 mg of calcium in her daily diet will absorb about 30% of that (300 mg), and that she will be losing that amount in her urine or from other sites, in sweat, for example, so that, overall, she is neither gaining nor losing any calcium from her body.

When pregnant, a woman needs to find some way to absorb extra dietary calcium from her diet or release calcium from her bones in order to obtain the 200 to 300 mg of calcium needed daily for her fetus. What actually occurs is that pregnant women increase the efficiency with which they absorb calcium from their diet. This increased absorbed calcium is the primary source of calcium for the fetus. Even more amazing is that this increase in calcium absorption occurs earlier in pregnancy than the fetus actually needs the extra calcium. It is a well thought out system for getting a fetus its calcium without robbing the mother of calcium for her own bones.

This increase occurs in part mediated by hormones, and in part due to more efficient conversion of vitamin D to its active form 1,25 dihydroxyvitamin D [$1,25(OH)_2D$]. A very thorough review of vitamin D during pregnancy and lactation was published in 2011 (Brannon and Picciano 2011). The authors indicate "a key physiologic change in pregnancy is the doubling of fractional calcium absorption" but they conclude with the idea "that vitamin D plays a role in this change is unlikely despite the association of similar temporal changes in serum $1,25(OH)_2D$ and calcium absorption." In other words, the active form of vitamin D increases during pregnancy, but available research studies, including those done in animals, seem to indicate that this increase in calcium absorption is not primarily due to vitamin D changes in pregnancy.

Overall, during pregnancy there is relatively little loss of calcium from the maternal skeleton. Pregnancy is not commonly associated with a large amount of maternal bone loss to meet the fetal needs, even in women with relatively low calcium intakes.

Lactation physiology

During lactation, however, the physiology is very different. The primary source of about 200 mg of calcium each day in breast milk is from the maternal skeleton, not from increases in maternal absorption of calcium. Urinary calcium losses go down somewhat during lactation, but there is still loss of calcium from the mother's skeleton. What is most fascinating about this is that after the baby is weaned, and a mother's menstrual periods have returned, she has a fairly rapid catch-up in her bone calcium content and bone mineral density (BMD). There is a general trend for women who have breast-fed to have a slightly greater, not lesser BMD than mothers who have formula-fed, although this difference is not large (Kalkwarf and Specker 2002; Hopkinson et al. 2000).

What is surprising to many people is that taking a lot of extra calcium during either pregnancy or lactation has little if any effect on this whole system. It is impossible to fundamentally prevent bone loss during lactation by taking extra calcium, and there is no additional calcium transferred to the fetus during pregnancy or to the infant from breast milk when an otherwise healthy woman takes either a calcium or vitamin D supplement. The system provides plenty of calcium to the fetus and infant without her needing to take in large amounts of calcium with no long-term effects on the mother.

There is no strong evidence for a role for high doses of vitamin D during lactation specific to the health of the mother or her infant. As discussed in Chapter 3, a dose of 6400 IU per day of vitamin D was shown in one small study to markedly increase the vitamin D content of mother's milk, but this is not physiologically necessary for maternal health, and vitamin D can be provided directly to the infant. High levels of vitamin D have not been shown to decrease maternal bone loss during lactation or to increase the bone mineralization of the infant.

Calcium and vitamin D in pregnancy and perinatal outcomes

Recently, attention has been paid to the possibility that vitamin D might be of value at high doses in improving pregnancy outcomes. This issue has been discussed widely in the media and in the medical literature. We would like to look at this more closely and reflect on how science is portrayed in the media related to this type of issue. First, however, we need to start with the role of *calcium* in determining pregnancy outcomes.

Over the last 20 years, there has been interest in the idea that calcium supplementation during pregnancy could decrease the risk of preterm delivery. A series of studies conducted mostly in developing countries suggested a markedly lower incidence of high blood pressure during pregnancy (pregnancy-induced hypertension), and a decreased risk of premature delivery related to the sequelae of this problem, called *pre-eclampsia*. These data remain fairly convincing in developing countries. A review of the data in 2011 continued to show strong evidence for such a benefit showing a 45% decreased risk in pregnancy-induced hypertension and a 30% decrease in all cause neonatal mortality (Imdad, Jabeen, and Bhutta 2011).

The initial data in the 1980s about this phenomenon were so compelling that in the United States, a large trial of calcium supplementation during pregnancy was conducted. Unfortunately, like many trials of nutritional interventions using supplements, this large study, which cost in the tens of millions of dollars, did not find an overall benefit to calcium supplementation in American women. This was a huge disappointment to say the least (Levine et al. 1997).

Resolving the discrepancy between the large U.S. trial and the international studies has been challenging. There is a consensus that calcium may be most beneficial, or only beneficial, in the highest risk populations such as are common in developing countries, or in women who have very low calcium intakes. For now, in the United States, there is agreement that providing the Recommended Dietary Allowance (RDA) intakes of calcium for pregnant women is important but there is no reason to recommend using high-dose supplements of calcium.

Let us turn to vitamin D and similar prenatal health care issues. A study published in 2007 suggested an association between very low vitamin D levels, such as serum 25(OH)D levels below about 12 ng/mL and the development of preeclampsia (Bodnar et al. 2007). Preventing or managing preeclampsia is a critical aspect of prenatal care and perinatal research. In the Bodnar study, women with preeclampsia had serum 25(OH)D levels below about 20 ng/mL. National data surveys in the United States show that about 28% of pregnant or lactating women in the United States have serum 25(OH)D levels below 20 ng/mL (Figure 7.1). Such a study is important as it suggests possible linkages between vitamin D and pregnancy outcome. As with calcium, vitamin D may be involved in blood pressure regulation, so an effect of vitamin D might be a real one.

However, studies showing such associations are only suggestive of an effect. There may have been many other reasons why women who developed preeclampsia had a lower vitamin D status. There are also concerns about the accuracy of the vitamin D levels that were done in those years due to problems with separating vitamin D_2 and vitamin D_3 in the analysis. This may or may not have had some effect on the results.

Much more attention was placed on this relationship between vitamin D and pregnancy outcome during 2010 and 2011. Data were presented at the annual meeting of pediatric scientists called the *Pediatric Academic Societies* in early May 2010 from a study conducted in South Carolina. It

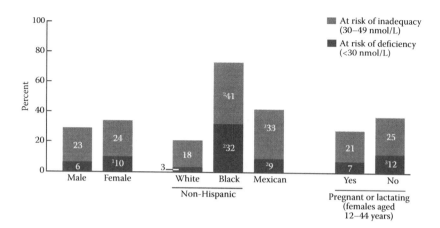

Figure 7.1 Age- and season-adjusted prevalence at risk of deficiency and inadequacy. Of note is that rates of low 25(OH)D values are not dissimilar between pregnancy and lactation, and other adult population groups. (From Looker AC, Johnson CL, Lacher DA, Pfeiffer CM, Schleicher RL, and Sempos CT, 2011, Vitamin D Status: United States, 2001–2006, *NCHS Data Brief*, March(59):1–8.)

was widely reported that this study showed that "taking vitamin D supplements during pregnancy is not only safe for mother and baby, but also can prevent preterm labor/births and infections." (*ScienceDaily*, May 2, 2010, http://www.sciencedaily.com/releases/2010/05/100501013417.htm)

Later that year, after a similar meeting of scientists in Europe in which these data were presented, the respected *Times of London* reported that "Powerful new evidence about the way that vitamin D can reduce the risk of premature births and boost the health of newborn babies has emerged from an international research conference in Bruges. Delegates were told that mothers who were given ten times the usual dose of vitamin D during pregnancy had their risk of premature birth reduced by half and had fewer small babies."

The scientist who presented this data was quoted in this article as saying, "I'm telling every pregnant mother I see to take 4,000 IUs and every nursing mother to take 6,400 IUs of vitamin D a day," and, "I think it is medical malpractice for obstetricians not to know what the vitamin D level of their patients is. This study will put them on notice" (*The Times of London*, October 10, 2009, http://www.timesonline.co.uk/tol/news/uk/scotland/article6868729.ece).

Now, before we examine the current science about this issue, let us stop to think about the implications of such a quote in the popular media. To the best of our knowledge, the author has never claimed to have been misquoted or retracted these quotes. It remains a prominent part of many online articles about vitamin D in pregnancy. The reader of these articles may not be made aware that the source of those quotes is not a physician and does not provide medical care for pregnant women. Therefore, if he is suggesting that he tells pregnant women and lactating women to take those high doses of vitamin D, he is doing so in his role as a scientist, not a physician.

The consequences of such quotes is concerning. Potentially, any woman who delivers a premature infant could threaten legal action against her obstetrician and claim that scientists have stated that this occurred because of a failure to test for vitamin D status as recommended by a leading scientist in the field. Notably, the Endocrine Society in 2010 and the American Academy of Pediatrics (AAP) in 2008 (Wagner, Greer, and AAP 2008) also recommend evaluation of maternal vitamin D status in pregnancy, although the AAP statement is more equivocal than is often quoted. It says "health-care professionals who provide obstetric care *should consider* assessing maternal vitamin D status by measuring the 25(OH)D concentrations of pregnant women" (italics added). The Endocrine Society did not suggest legal action might be taken against physicians who did not test for vitamin D during pregnancy.

Therefore, what is the actual evidence from the South Carolina pregnancy study and what do we know about vitamin D, preeclampsia and preterm delivery? Well, one big problem is that we do not know all the details about that study. The study was presented at meetings and with written abstracts. These are not, however, adequate for evaluation of a research study's results. The only way the medical and scientific community can evaluate research is via reviewing all of the results that are published in a peer-reviewed manuscript. A manuscript with partial results from this study in South Carolina was first made publicly available in the medical literature in June 2011 (Hollis et al. 2011).

In this study, a total of just fewer than 500 women were randomized to receive a supplement of 400 IU, 2000 IU, or 4000 IU of vitamin D daily beginning in the second trimester of pregnancy. According to the original study design, the primary outcomes of interest were to be:

1. Serum 25(OH)D levels throughout pregnancy and following delivery.
2. Bone mineral density of both mother and infant.

To find this information originally received by clinicaltrials.gov in February 2006, visit (accessed August 15, 2011) http://clinicaltrials.gov/ct2/show/study/NCT00292591 (most recent online update September 23, 2010).

Specific reference to risk of preterm delivery or preeclampsia was not part of the original study protocol nor was the sample size of patients who needed to be enrolled in the study to identify a biologically meaningful effect of vitamin D therapy on these outcomes calculated for such endpoints.

When reviewing this manuscript from the study in South Carolina, an initial concern was that the authors clearly state that they have additional results from the study that were not published in the article. It is not clear what those results were or if the second primary outcome related to bone mineral density was ever completed. This is problematic in that they concluded the article, stating as they have in interviews and public presentations that:

> These findings suggest that the current vitamin D Estimated Average Requirement [EAR] and RDA for pregnant women issued in 2010 by the Institute of Medicine [IOM] should be raised to 4000 IU vitamin D per day so that all women regardless of race attain optimal nutritional and hormonal vitamin D status throughout pregnancy. (Hollis et al. 2011)

This statement is considerably different from recent recommendations from the IOM (2011) and even the Endocrine Society (Holick et al. 2011). When interpreting and understanding it, the first problem is that the authors recommend that the EAR and RDA be the same value. Using the correct terms in criticizing the IOM recommendations would be helpful and make it easier to understand the authors' perspective. The EAR and the RDA, as described in Chapter 2, are completely different terms and suggesting that both terms should be the same represents a lack of understanding of the terms and of the current way in which the IOM present dietary recommendations.

In brief, the EAR and the RDA have different meanings. The EAR for vitamin D of 400 IU per day during pregnancy represents a recommendation most relevant to population *groups*. It is a value at which about 50% of individuals meet their requirements. The RDA of 600 IU per day during pregnancy is an intake recommendation more useful for evaluating an *individual's* diet and reflects intakes that meet the needs of 97.5% of the population.

Once one can agree on the indicators for an *optimal* serum 25(OH) D value, dose-response and population distribution data can be used to derive estimates of the EAR and subsequently the RDA based on this value. Specifically, in the Hollis et al. (2011) report, about half of mothers achieved a serum 25(OH)D level of about 32 ng/mL with a supplement of 400 IU per day. This is twice the current target serum 25(OH)D value for determining the EAR of 16 ng/mL. Therefore, this means that even if one believes that a serum 25(OH)D level of 32 ng/mL provides health benefits in pregnancy, the IOM got it right with their EAR of 400 IU per day. Well, it is a bit trickier than that because there is a difference between supplement dose and total vitamin D dietary intake, but even then, it would be pretty close using the IOM values.

The more important question to ask is this: Is it necessary to target a serum 25(OH)D of at least 32 ng/mL for the RDA during pregnancy or in newborn infants rather than the 20 ng/mL value set by the IOM?

The Hollis et al. (2011) report provides data showing an increase in the urinary calcium:creatinine ratio (Ca:Cr) with higher serum 25(OH)D levels that according to the authors *appears* to *normalize* at about 30 ng/mL. The problem with this Ca:Cr description is that it is not clear why this is important or is evidence of improved health outcomes. First of all, no statistical analysis of this conclusion is provided and the graph does not clearly show this value *normalizing* or *maximizing* at 30 ng/mL. Furthermore, there is no evidence at all that the Ca:Cr ratio has to be normalized or that normalizing it makes any difference in pregnancy outcome.

Although a low Ca:Cr ratio has been associated with preeclampsia in a few small studies, there is no evidence from controlled trials of a decrease in preeclampsia with supplemental vitamin D (or even calcium) to increase the Ca:Cr ratio. There is not an established definition of a normal urine Ca:Cr ratio related to biological outcomes in the second and third trimester of pregnancy. The study also only obtained a randomly timed Ca:Cr ratio in an unfasted state. A fasted value or better yet, a 24-hour total urine calcium would be much better to assess urinary calcium excretion. In general, Ca:Cr values are of limited value and may not identify risks or benefits of either calcium or vitamin D supplementation in any population. Notably, the Ca:Cr ratio was not part of the original study design as a key outcome measure.

Additionally, although the authors found a higher value of the active form of vitamin D, $1,25(OH)_2D$ with higher doses of vitamin D supplementation, there is no evidence for any targeted value of $1,25(OH)_2D$, related to clinical maternal or neonatal outcomes or evidence that maximizing $1,25(OH)_2D$ has specific health benefits. In fact, it is very unlikely based on available animal data that this is true, and there are no efforts in any population of healthy individuals to target high $1,25(OH)_2D$ levels.

The authors further comment upon the optimization of calcium absorption at a serum level of 25(OH)D of 32 ng/mL. This value, however, is not established in pregnancy, and calcium absorption efficiency is optimized at much lower 25(OH)D levels in large studies involving older children and adolescents as we described in Chapter 6. Whether 32 ng/mL is a valid target for optimizing calcium absorption in nonpregnant women remains highly controversial. Finally, no data exist relating a range of neonatal 25(OH)D levels to calcium absorption efficiency (Chapter 3). Clinical evidence of vitamin D deficiency has not been shown for serum 25(OH)D values above approximately 10 to 12 ng/mL in neonates and young infants.

Related to infant outcomes, data in the tables of the Hollis et al. (2011) paper indicates that there were no statistically significant differences in infant and maternal outcomes for the frequency of Cesarean sections, birth weight, gestational age, or need for Neonatal Intensive Care Unit (NICU) admission based on vitamin D supplementation dose. Recall that none of these were listed as primary outcomes of the study in the original study descriptions. Developing such outcomes after a study is over is fraught with the possibility of biases and is generally considered of only limited value in hypothesis development for further studies.

From a safety perspective, it was reassuring that no complications were seen in the women who completed this study. However, this finding also needs to be interpreted with caution. As noted by the authors, they evaluated supplementation only during the second and third trimesters of pregnancy. Therefore, recommendations and safety considerations for the entirety of pregnancy are premature. The study had the possibility for multiple biases related to safety as well. The randomization as required by the Institutional Review Board (IRB) prevented those with high baseline serum 25(OH)D values from receiving the highest supplement dose. Furthermore, several women with high serum 25(OH)D levels were taken off of supplementation during the study.

Even more concerning is that over 100 of the women who started the study did not finish it. The overall small sample size, high-dropout rates, and withdrawal rates are not proof of safety for the entire population of pregnant women in the United States. The final sample size for all three groups combined was about 350 women. This small sample size that would account for 0.3% of pregnant women would be unlikely to find the occurrence of a complication. Only about 120 women got the 4000 IU per day dose. If that dose caused a complication in 1:200 women (0.5%) for example, there is a good chance it would have been missed. Multiply 0.5% by 4 million pregnancies in the United States each year and you get about 20,000 pregnancies. This is hardly adequate or compelling proof of safety.

Therefore, let us look at the evidence. There is only one small controlled trial of high-dose vitamin D supplementation in pregnancy (Hollis et al. 2011). It found no benefits currently published to outcomes for the infants at or after birth and limited evidence of safety in the mothers. Based on this study, where does the idea come from that this should be a global recommendation for all women? Should obstetricians really be at risk for being sued if they do not monitor vitamin D levels in pregnancy?

For mothers: Make your own decisions with the advice of your obstetrician, midwife, or other caregiver. For everyone: Read the literature critically and consider editorial commentary about these data (Abrams 2011). We should reflect carefully on how we wish to spend our limited resources to provide care for our population. Not every test that can be done should be done, even during pregnancy.

Teenage pregnancy and lactation

First of all, for the most part, it would be best if teenagers did not have babies. However, those of us working in pediatrics and especially in neonatology are aware that this does happen, and it is important to investigate and understand the consequences for the bone health of teenagers having a baby, especially those less than about 16 years of age.

Recall that the peak time for bone mineral accumulation in teenage girls is right before menarche, the first menstrual period. The period of rapid bone growth in adolescent girls begins at least 2 years before menarche and has slowed down considerably by 2 years after menarche. Therefore, for the most part, except for girls who become pregnant prior to 15 or 16 years of age, most of their own growth and bone mineralization is nearly, but not fully complete.

However, some increase in bone mineralization occurs in young adults throughout adolescence, with a gradual reaching of peak bone mass in females in the late 20s, although a value nearly equal to peak bone mass is achieved by about age 18 or so. Therefore, any teenage pregnancy may have some affect on maternal bone mineralization and achievement of peak bone mass, even if the biggest effect would be for those less than about 16 years of age.

There are relatively few studies evaluating this group of girls related to their bone health. As one can imagine, they are not the easiest group to identify early in pregnancy (or before pregnancy!) and with whom to conduct longitudinal studies during pregnancy and lactation.

One study identified low serum 25(OH)D levels in pregnant teens with about half of the teens having levels less than 20 ng/mL. However, the consequences of these low vitamin D levels was uncertain as pregnancy outcomes were not included in the report (Davis et al. 2010). Another small study suggested that fetal bone growth was affected by very low calcium intake in pregnant African-American adolescents, but long-term follow-up was not provided (Chang et al. 2003).

Although some early data raised concerns about lactation during adolescence and maternal bone loss, this has not been found in more recent studies. A review of this topic in 2005 found no evidence for an effect on maternal bone health (Ward, Adams, and Mughal 2005). However, more research is needed in this area. It is important to remember that the RDA for calcium during pregnancy or lactation for someone who is less than 19 years of age is 1300 mg per day, the same as for any other adolescent.

Taken on the whole, it is almost certain that the benefits of breast-feeding to both the mother and the infant of adolescent mothers is vastly greater than any possible effect on maternal bone mineralization from breast-feeding. Adolescent mothers who are breast-feeding need to discuss contraception options carefully with their health-care provider.

Although exclusive breast-feeding decreases the likelihood of a further pregnancy, it is not perfect and many of these mothers may not exclusively breast-feed.

Teamwork in Medicine

We work at Texas Children's Hospital, a large pediatric hospital in Houston, Texas (www.texaschildrenshospital.org). Our children's hospital has partnered with its affiliated medical school, Baylor College of Medicine, (www.bcm.edu) and its affiliated Department of Pediatrics and Department of Obstetrics and Gynecology to open a very large new perinatal center (http://vision2010.texaschildrens.org/maternity_building.html). Now, we are proud of this new center, but the reason we mention it here is that it represents a real merging of the fields of obstetrics and neonatology with the goal of seamlessly integrating the care of the highest risk infants between the obstetrician and the pediatric caregivers, including the neonatologists.

Not long ago these fields were very separate. Symbolically and practically, when the umbilical cord was cut, the baby was handed over to the pediatrician or neonatologist and the division of responsibilities was clear.

Those familiar with the space shuttle missions, which sadly have ended, might be aware of the transfer of responsibility between Kennedy Space Center in Florida and Johnson Space Center in Houston seconds after the shuttle launches when it cleared the control tower. This precise transfer of control was often noted by the mission launch commentators with the words "Houston controlling." Of course, teamwork between the two sites was crucial throughout the launch process, but there was a clear delineation of mission control at a specified time in the flight.

In medicine, such transfers also occur but they are complex. Patients are transferred within and between hospitals, and care is transferred between doctors, nurses, and other caregivers. New guidelines restricting the number of consecutive hours that physicians-in-training can work has led to even more transfers of responsibilities each day within teaching hospitals.

The possibilities for error during patient transfers and medical team transfer of care are tremendous, and much effort and thought has gone into trying to make sure such handoffs are done in a collaborative way. In terms of neonatology and obstetrics, this has become a major focus. Whenever a mother is pregnant with a baby with a probable major congenital problem, a multidisciplinary team is assembled to discuss the problem and plan for the *in utero*, delivery, and postdelivery management.

For example, when a baby is found to have a congenital heart problem during a prenatal ultrasound, then the mother and baby are referred to our perinatal team for evaluation. This evaluation includes visits with a pediatric cardiologist, high-risk obstetrician, and a neonatologist. Parents are invited to tour the appropriate hospital areas where their baby will receive care. After the initial ultrasounds and fetal cardiac echos are reviewed, the case is reviewed before a team of doctors, nurses, social workers, and others involved in managing the infant and the pregnancy. Discussions are held that may include ethical issues and practical issues related to the initial care of the infant.

This is teamwork in medicine at a level rarely seen until very recently. Implicit in this approach is an understanding that what the obstetrician does for the patient affects how the neonatologist handles the infant, which, in turn, affects what the pediatric cardiologist does for the newborn, and so forth. None of these doctors work in a vacuum, they are not Dr. House, and none work effectively unless the other aspects of care, including nursing, dietetic, social work, and spiritual care, are properly in place and linked to the team.

References

Abrams SA. 2011. Vitamin D supplementation during pregnancy. *J Bone Miner Res.* 26:2338–40. Editorials are short opportunities to respond and comment upon important research papers. In this editorial, a few of the flaws in the idea that women need 4000 IU daily of vitamin D based on a single research study are discussed in a way similar to this chapter. Draw your own conclusions. (Not free online.)

Bodnar LM, Catov JM, Simhan HN, Holick MF, Powers RW, and Roberts JM. 2007. Maternal vitamin D deficiency increases the risk of preeclampsia. *J Clin Endocrinol Metab* 92:3517–22. Association is not causation. It is not surprising that women with low 25(OH)D levels are more likely to have a range of complications in their pregnancy. This may be due to race, lifestyle factors, or a whole range of dietary issues which are reflected in the 25(OH)D level. A simple multiple regression or attempt to do covariate analysis is imperfect in dealing with this broad range of covariates. Regardless, this association should be tested with a controlled trial. (Free online.)

Brannon PM, and Picciano MF. 2011. Vitamin D in pregnancy and lactation in humans. *Annu Rev Nutr* 31:89–115. This is the view that doubts the current data to support a need for high-dose vitamin D supplementation. Dr. Picciano, who spent her career working in the area of dietary supplementation, died in 2010. (Visit http://nutrition.psu.edu/news/newsletter_Fall2010/memoriam.html to read about Dr. Picciano.) (Not free online.)

Chang SC, O'Brien KO, Nathanson MS, Caulfield LE, Mancini J, and Witter FR. 2003. Fetal femur length is influenced by maternal dairy intake in pregnant African-American adolescents. *Am J Clin Nutr* 77:1248–54. This is a small study suggesting that very low ma…nal calcium intakes might be associated with lower bone growth in the fetus. Long-term follow-up would have been helpful to know if this was a real phenomenon. (Free online.)

Davis LM, Chang SC, Mancini J, Nathanson MS, Witter FR, and O'Brien KO. 2010. Vitamin D insufficiency is prevalent among pregnant African-American adolescents. *J Pediatr Adolesc Gynecol* 23:45–52. It is not unexpected that this group would have low vitamin D levels. It is far from clear that these levels are directly related to pregnancy outcomes, but this should be evaluated in controlled supplementation trials. However, conducting a controlled supplementation trial beginning in early pregnancy in teenagers would be extremely difficult. (Not free online.)

Holick MF, Binkley NC, Bischoff-Ferrari HA, Gordon CM, Hanley DA, Heaney RP, Murad MH, and Weaver CM. 2011. Evaluation, treatment, and prevention of vitamin D deficiency: An endocrine society clinical practice guideline. *J Clin Endocrinol Metab* 96:1911–30. See annotation in Chapter 2 "References." (Not free online.)

Hollis BW, Johnson D, Hulsey TC, Ebeling M, and Wagner CL. 2011. Vitamin D supplementation during pregnancy: Double blind, randomized clinical trial of safety and effectiveness. *J Bone Miner Res* 26:2741–57. A detailed description of this study is in this chapter. It is a limited study needing much more confirmation before being useful in establishing DRI values in pregnancy or establishing further public policy recommendations. (Not free online.)

Hopkinson JM, Butte NF, Ellis K, and Smith EO. 2000. Lactation delays postpartum bone mineral accretion and temporarily alters its regional distribution in women. *J Nutr* 130:777–83. Mothers lose bone during lactation but get it back after weaning. Possibly even with a bonus amount! In no way should mothers be concerned that if they are otherwise healthy and have a normal diet that lactation poses a long-term risk of osteoporosis. Whether there is a decrease in osteoporosis in women based on lactation remains somewhat uncertain, with an overall slight trend in the literature to support this idea to a limited degree. Further studies are needed. (Free online.)

Imdad A, Jabeen A, and Bhutta ZA. 2011. Role of calcium supplementation during pregnancy in reducing risk of developing gestational hypertensive disorders: A meta-analysis of studies from developing countries. *BMC Public Health* 11 Suppl 3:S18. This is a review demonstrating a large benefit in developing countries to providing calcium supplementation during pregnancy. However, implementation is a major problem. (Free online.)

Institute of Medicine. 2011. *Dietary Reference Intakes for Calcium and Vitamin D*. Washington, DC: National Academy Press. See annotation in Chapter 2 "References."

Kalkwarf HJ, and Specker BL. 2002. Bone mineral changes during pregnancy and lactation. *Endocrine* 17:49–53. Having babies does not affect long-term risk of osteoporosis. Neither does breast-feeding them. On the whole, it is more likely that long-term breast-feeding is good for the mother's health in many respects than any concerns that the milk has any long-term negative effects on the maternal skeleton. (Not free online.)

Levine RJ, Hauth JC, Curet LB, Sibai BM, Catalano PM, Morris CD, DerSimonian R, Esterlitz JR, Raymond EG, Bild DE, Clemens JD, and Cutler JA. 1997. Trial of calcium to prevent preeclampsia. *N Engl J Med* 337:69–76. It does not work. At least calcium supplementation did not work to decrease preeclampsia and preterm birth in the United States among women with normal calcium intakes. However, there was some suggestion even in these data of a benefit for pregnancy outcomes among women with low calcium intakes. In developing countries, there is much stronger evidence for an effect in populations with usual low calcium intakes. Numerous research studies are underway to evaluate how best to translate the results in developing countries into a practical plan. (Not free online.)

Ward KA, Adams JE, and Mughal MZ. 2005. Bone status during adolescence, pregnancy and lactation. *Curr Opin Obstet Gynecol* 17:435–9. There is no evidence that teenagers harm their bones during pregnancy or lactation. This does not mean that teenage pregnancy is a good idea. But, teenage mothers usually should be encouraged to breast-feed without major concern about maternal bone health. They should also be counseled carefully about forms of contraception to be used that support breast-feeding but will keep them from becoming teenage mothers of two children. (Not free online.)

Wagner CL, Greer FR, and American Academy of Pediatrics (AAP), Section on Breastfeeding and Committee on Nutrition. 2008. Prevention of rickets and vitamin D deficiency in infants, children, and adolescents. *Pediatrics* 122(5):1142–52 [published correction appears in *Pediatrics* 2009; 123(1):197]. See annotation in Chapter 2 "References." (Free online.)

chapter eight

Children with chronic illnesses

For bones to grow in children, lots of things have to happen in the right sequence. In children with chronic illnesses, a lot can go wrong with this sequence. This description is not complete, but is a start to help families and caregivers understand the process.

1. Forming new bone requires a normally developed bone structure, sometimes called *bone architecture*. This requires normal bone growth and normal bone protein to develop the matrix that is mineralized primarily by calcium and phosphorus. Abnormalities related to genetic causes include osteogenesis imperfecta, protein insufficiency (malnutrition), or other genetic conditions such as many chromosome disorders. Rare conditions or nutritional deficiencies including vitamin C and zinc deficiency can also alter the structure of bone. There has been relatively little research in this topic. For the most part, genetic abnormalities of bone do not respond well to nutritional interventions.

2. The bone minerals must be absorbed and carried to the growing bone. That is, the intestine must be functioning normally both to allow adequate absorption of nutrients and prevent excessive loss of nutrients. Many chronic illnesses in children are associated with abnormalities of mineral absorption or excess loss of minerals in the urine and stool. An example of this would be children with inflammatory bowel diseases such as Crohn's disease.

3. The kidneys must be working both to form active vitamin D and to prevent bone mineral loss. Furthermore, severe renal failure poses a problem in which the body is unable to excrete phosphorus. Diets given to children, even very small infants with renal failure, are therefore low in calcium and phosphorus leading to a greater risk of poor bone mineralization.

4. The endocrine system must be functioning normally to allow for growth hormone, estrogen, thyroid hormone, and other bone-related hormones to be released. There must not be an excess of some hormones either because that can cause hyperthyroidism, for example. Eating disorders can lead to abnormalities in the endocrine system needed for bone growth.

5. The diet must contain sufficient calcium and phosphorus and the individual must have an adequate vitamin D status. In any number of conditions, there may be an inadequate nutrient intake. Some of these are not obvious. For example, babies with congenital heart disease or chronic lung disease are often limited in the volume of feedings they can tolerate without worsening their heart failure. As such, they may have trouble achieving a full intake of minerals as would be ingested by a healthy infant.

6. Medications that can negatively affect bone or diet need to be recognized. Some antiseizure medications affect vitamin D or other aspects of bone mineral metabolism. Steroid therapy affects many aspects of the bone mineralization process, and in both adults and children can be a major cause of bone demineralization and fractures. For the most part, this effect is relatively limited in those who are only using inhaled steroids for asthma, for example (Turpeinin et al. 2010). Chemotherapy drugs may harm nutrient absorption or increase secretion. Some medications can also decrease appetite causing a poor dietary intake.

However, due to the wonderful advances in health care for children, we now have many children who survive very long term with conditions including cystic fibrosis, leukemia, severe cerebral palsy, and intestinal failure (Abrams 2011). Each of these conditions and many more has profound implications for bone health and potentially for diet and growth. It is impossible for a book like this to do justice to every chronic illness in children and adolescents. However, we would like to consider a few specific conditions as examples.

Three conditions we will specifically consider are juvenile arthritis, leukemia, and cystic fibrosis. Each of these reflects some of the challenges in optimizing bone health in children with chronic illnesses. Research is ongoing into bone health in these conditions, but clear recommendations are not yet available. Our descriptions here are meant to illustrate principles of evaluation and bone health-related management, not provide specific guidance for individuals with these or other conditions.

The nutritional guidelines of the Institute of Medicine (IOM) related to calcium and vitamin D (IOM 2011), as well as the position statements of the American Academy of Pediatrics (AAP), and other organizations related to mineral needs in healthy children do not usually relate specifically to children with chronic illnesses. Some organizations, such as the Endocrine Society (Holick et al. 2011), have included comments related to specific disease conditions, although these generally are not provided specific to pediatric populations. When organizations publish specific guidelines related to various chronic health conditions, they do not usually use the Dietary Reference Intake (DRI) framework or include specific values such as the Recommended Dietary Allowance (RDA). Sometimes, these guidelines were developed by experts in the disease with or without substantial input from nutritional experts. Many times, recommendations come in the form of suggestions for high-dose therapy without details of monitoring or desired outcome.

For example, consider the situation of liver (hepatobiliary) disease in children. The North American Society for Pediatric Gastroenterology, Hepatology and Nutrition (NASPGHAN) states that "large doses of vitamin D may be needed to correct osteomalacia (rickets)" (http://www.naspghan.org/wmspage.cfm?parm1=128). The doses they suggest of 1.25 to 5 mg per day are equal to 50,000 to 200,000 IU per day (where 1 mg of vitamin D is 40,000 IU). These doses are, to say the least, very large and orders of magnitude above the Upper Limit (UL) for healthy children for vitamin D. As such, very careful monitoring for safety would be needed with these doses. Caregivers would need to carefully consider which children exactly needed these types of doses and for how long they were needed.

Having said that, there are still very few guidelines about nutrition and bone health in children with chronic illnesses. Generally, such guidelines recommend following the RDA for healthy children or give recommendations to provide calcium, or more recently, vitamin D supplementation at an often-arbitrary amount. As this field develops further, it is worthwhile to return to some of the physiology we discussed before and consider how it applies to children with chronic illnesses, using the examples of juvenile arthritis, leukemia, and cystic fibrosis.

Juvenile arthritis

Juvenile arthritis and related rheumatological conditions have long been known to be associated with decreased bone mineral and the potential for increased fractures. Almost half of children with juvenile arthritis will have bone mineral content (BMC) below normal during early adulthood (Lien et al. 2003).

First, children with severe forms of juvenile arthritis are often treated with medications that interfere with calcium absorption and bone formation. These include systemic steroids and medications such as methotrexate (Thornton et al. 2011). The use of these medications can have a profound and life-long effect on bone mineral, especially in the early course of the illness. There is inadequate research on important topics like the dosage and forms of steroids that have an effect on bone mineral metabolism in children. It is also likely that children with juvenile arthritis and related conditions also have abnormalities in bone mineralization related to overall poorer diet and slow linear growth. Some of this is related to their medications but it may not be entirely medication related.

In treating children with juvenile arthritis and related conditions, it is reasonable to ask whether any specialized testing or therapy is needed related to bone health. Although guidance for this is variable, there is no obvious reason that dietary intake of calcium above the RDA levels is necessary or helpful in most cases. In those conditions with a high level of malabsorption, such as inflammatory bowel disease, this may be different. Nonetheless, many caregivers choose to increase the intake of nutrients in chronic illnesses including juvenile arthritis.

Increasing nutrient intakes may or may not be helpful. However, caution should be used in increasing intakes of calcium or vitamin D above the tolerable upper intake level. There is even a small study in which 2000 IU per day of vitamin D along with calcium had no benefit in improving bone mineralization in children with juvenile arthritis (Hillman et al. 2008). Exceeding the UL, especially by a large amount, should only be done in the context of clinical trials with safety monitoring, or in individuals with careful monitoring for toxicity by the caregivers.

Leukemia

Childhood cancer and treatments for leukemia can have adverse effects on bone health. The reasons for bone health morbidity are multifactorial, including the disease process itself, chemotherapy, irradiation of endocrine organs, poor nutrition, genetic predisposition, inactivity, and delayed puberty. These factors can lead to decreased BMC, increased fracture risk, osteopenia, failure to attain peak bone mass, and predisposition to osteoporosis later in life.

Recent data suggests this may affect up to half of all long-term survivors of Acute Lymphocytic Leukemia (ALL) and lead to very long-term risks of osteoporosis (Benmiloud et al. 2010). More research is needed to determine how best to both prevent this bone loss during cancer treatment and to assist in catch-up for mineral losses later in childhood and adolescence. The wonderful progress that has been made in treating children with cancer, especially ALL, must now lead to further research to determine the best ways to care for them throughout their life.

There is minimal data relating cancer in children to vitamin D status or treatment. Although literally hundreds of such studies, with frequently conflicting and controversial results exist in the literature related to adults, essentially nothing is known related to this in children. This is unfortunate and partly related to the challenge of convincing funding organizations of the need to focus research efforts on nutrition in children with cancer both during their treatment and throughout their growing years.

Cystic fibrosis

Optimizing bone health in children and young adults with cystic fibrosis has several of the same challenges as it does for children with juvenile arthritis, but some unique ones as well. Because the condition is inherently associated with fat malabsorption, vitamin D may not be adequately absorbed from the diet or supplements. Therefore, it is common and reasonable to routinely monitor serum 25(OH)D levels in children with cystic fibrosis. What is more controversial is whether there is any benefit to achieving a high serum 25(OH)D level ng/mL, such as one above 30 ng/mL, and what approach should be used for increasing serum 25(OH)D levels when standard vitamin supplementation is inadequate.

These issues remain controversial, but at present, there is no evidence from controlled trials indicating that achieving any specific serum 25(OH)D level above that recommended for children who do not have cystic fibrosis is necessary for bone health in children with cystic fibrosis. Neither extremely high-dose vitamin D nor calcium supplements are of proven benefit for these children. Recommendations to use suntan beds or similar approaches should be viewed with concern and done in the context of controlled clinical trials. A recent *Cochrane Review* did not find evidence of a benefit from vitamin D supplementation, although the data were considered very limited (Ferguson and Chang 2009).

As with other conditions, there is very little scientific evidence to guide clinicians in how best to manage bone mineral deficiency in children and young adults with cystic fibrosis. Very long-term studies are needed beginning in infancy and early childhood. However, it can be challenging to conduct such studies due to the challenge of identifying and matching these children with children who are similar in growth but do not have any chronic illnesses.

Summary related to bone health and chronic illnesses

Every disease has unique risk factors for bone health in children. In general, it is uncommon that inadequate dietary calcium or vitamin D intake is the major problem related to bone health in children with chronic conditions. The reverse is also true; giving more calcium and vitamin D is no guarantee of a fix for bone health problems in children with chronic illnesses.

Each child needs an individual evaluation based on disease physiology and severity, Dual-Energy X-ray Absorptiometry (DXA) findings, and appropriate lab tests. A comprehensive diet evaluation by a registered dietitian for multivitamin/multimineral supplements may be better than a limited targeting of calcium and/or vitamin D. Careful consideration needs to also be made about the target goal. Fixing biochemical numbers may not be as important as enhancing long-term growth. Sometimes, the disease or its therapy (e.g., steroids) will lead to poor bone growth for a while, with the opportunity for catch-up later. Consultation with an expert in the individual disease and its bone manifestations is critical.

There is extremely little research into this area in children. Those groups who support research into disease therapy should strongly encourage further well-conducted physiological studies of pediatric diseases and nutrition, including bone health. Controlled trials are important, but some animal, basic science, and physiological studies such as determining mineral absorption in different circumstances are needed as well.

The Medical Home: Providing Comprehensive Pediatric Care for Children with Chronic Illnesses

It is no secret that medicine, especially in the United States, is at a crossroads where many decisions must be made about who provides what forms of health care to individuals, including children with chronic illnesses. It is reasonable to ask how the community-based general pediatrician fits into long-term care plans for such children. After all, whether it is an infant with congenital heart disease in the midst of multiple surgeries in the early years of life, or a teenager with cerebral palsy, care must be apportioned that considers both the unique aspects of the disease process and the general needs of health care for infants, children, and adolescents.

One approach to this is the idea of the medical home, or, in this case, the pediatric home, which is described in this free online article (http://pediatrics.aappublications.org/content/127/4/604.full). What does this mean? Take a look at this Web site from the AAP (http://www.pediatricmedhome.org/). This is a site for pediatricians to develop their practice as a medical home. Some of what is there is for pediatricians who have registered with the Web site group, but other very interesting ideas are public (http://www.pediatricmedhome.org/qib/). The goal is to develop pediatricians and their staff to truly understand the idea of comprehensive care for children, especially those with chronic illnesses, and to establish practical approaches to management and organization of such care that are community-based and reflect a full use of all available resources.

It is an understatement that any family that has a child with special needs has been very frustrated by the disorganization and complexity of putting together resources for their child's care. It is crucial to try to identify a pediatric medical home for children with special needs.

References

Abrams SA. 2011. "Osteopenia and Bone Health in Patients with Intestinal Failure." In *Clinical Management of Intestinal Failure*, edited by Duggan C, Gura KM, and Jaksic T. Boca Raton, FL: CRC Press. A review of bone health issues especially in children who have intestinal failure. (Not free online.)

Benmiloud S, Steffens M, Beauloye V, de Wandeleer A, Devogelaer JP, Brichard B, Vermylen C, and Maiter D. 2010. Long-term effects on bone mineral density of different therapeutic schemes for acute lymphoblastic leukemia or nonHodgkin lymphoma during childhood. *Horm Res Paediatr* 74:241–50. Authors conclude that low bone mass is frequently observed in adult survivors of childhood leukemia and Hodgkin's lymphoma, especially in boys. (Not free online.)

Ferguson JH and Chang AB. 2009. Vitamin D supplementation for cystic fibrosis. *Cochrane Database Syst Rev* October 7;(4):CD007298. Not much evidence for any benefit to high-dose supplementation. Well-performed controlled trials are needed. (Not free online.)

Hillman LS, Cassidy JT, Chanetsa F, Hewett JE, Higgins BJ, and Robertson JD. 2008. Percent true calcium absorption, mineral metabolism, and bone mass in children with arthritis: Effect of supplementation with vitamin D_3 and calcium. *Arthritis Rheum* 58:3255–63. No real effect of vitamin D or calcium supplementation on bone mineral mass in children with arthritis. Few pay adequate attention to such *negative* studies and they get little media attention. (Free online.)

Holick MF, Binkley NC, Bischoff-Ferrari HA, Gordon CM, Hanley DA, Heaney RP, Murad MH, and Weaver CM. 2011. Evaluation, treatment, and prevention of vitamin D deficiency: An endocrine society clinical practice guideline. *J Clin Endocrinol Metab* 96:1911–30. See Chapter 2 for a detailed description of this report. (Not free online.)

Institute of Medicine. 2011. *Dietary Reference Intakes for Calcium and vitamin D*. Washington, DC: National Academy Press. See annotation in Chapter 2 "References."

Lien G, Flatø B, Haugen M, Vinje O, Sørskaar D, Dale K, Johnston V, Egeland T, and Førre Ø. 2003. Frequency of osteopenia in adolescents with early-onset juvenile idiopathic arthritis: A long-term outcome study of one hundred five patients. *Arthritis Rheum* 48:2214–23. Osteopenia occurs in about 40% of adolescents with juvenile arthritis. (Free online.)

Thornton J, Pye SR, O'Neill TW, Rawlings D, Francis RM, Symmons DP, Ashcroft DM, and Foster HE. 2011. Bone health in adult men and women with a history of juvenile idiopathic arthritis. *J Rheumatol* 38:1689–93. Juvenile arthritis can have an effect on bone mineral density that persists into adulthood. (Not free online.)

Turpeinen M, Pelkonen AS, Nikander K, Sorva R, Selroos O, Juntunen-Backman K, and Haahtela T. 2010. Bone mineral density in children treated with daily or periodical inhaled budesonide: The Helsinki early intervention childhood asthma study. *Pediatr Res* 68:169–73. A complex well-controlled trial of the effects of inhaled steroids on bone mineral density. The conclusions were that daily dosing during early puberty had a small, but significant effect on bones and height, whereas intermittent dosing did not. (Not free online.)

chapter nine

Myths and realities of calcium intake in children

Can't we just fortify all our foods?

So far we have focused on an age-based approach to bone health. It is worthwhile to consider a few issues that we have not discussed in detail related to calcium that cross age boundaries and are of importance.

We will begin by discussing a bit more about sources of calcium in the diet. Figure 9.1 shows calcium intakes based on age and race or ethnicity in the United States. In Figure 9.2, the overall data are shown compared to the Estimated Average Requirement (EAR) at each age. In general, it is clear that children age 1 to 8 years have average intakes at or well above the EAR whereas this is not true for adolescents, especially girls.

In the United States, dairy products provide about 60% of the calcium that children receive. Furthermore, dairy is a source of highly bioavailable calcium. Soy beverages and some vegetables, especially spinach, contain calcium, but those forms are not as bioavailable as the calcium found in dairy foods. That is, the oxalate in spinach, for example, almost completely blocks dietary absorption of calcium. Limited data similarly indicates that calcium from soymilk is absorbed somewhat less than that from cow's milk, although this is somewhat controversial.

What is clear is that there are many myths about dairy products that need to be addressed. Going through all of these would be too much for this book, but here are a few brief comments.

1. *Myth*: Some believe that chocolate milk does not have absorbable calcium. *Reality*: This is based on some very old research. Chocolate milk has calcium that is well absorbed. It is important that we continue to work for lower calorie chocolate milk, but, from a calcium perspective, absorption from chocolate milk is not a problem. More about chocolate milk can be found in the Chapter 15 "Frequently Asked Questions."

2. *Myth*: African Americans cannot have any dairy products. *Reality*: Children with lactose intolerance, including African Americans, can often tolerate some dairy products including lactose-free milk and

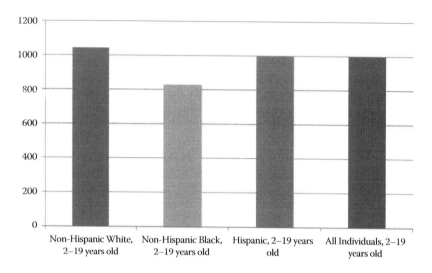

Figure 9.1 Calcium consumption in the United States based on age, race, and ethnicity. (Individuals 2 years and over [excluding pregnant and/or lactating females and breast-fed children], day 1 food and supplement intake data, weighted.) (From NHANES 2005–2006, "What We Eat in America," Washington, DC: U.S. Department of Agriculture, Agricultural Research Service.)

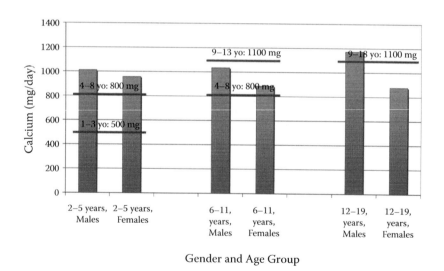

Figure 9.2 Comparison of calcium intakes with the 2011 EAR values from the IOM based on age groups.

some cheeses. It is not true that African-American children all have severe lactose intolerance and cannot have any dairy in their diet.

3. *Myth*: Milk makes a teenager gain weight. *Reality*: Milk does not make adolescents or most anyone else gain weight when it is low-fat milk provided as part of a healthy diet. This is a complex issue and science is ongoing in relation to it. On the whole, however, milk consumption does not lead to weight gain and may be very helpful in weight maintenance. There is highly conflicting evidence about a role for dairy products or calcium supplementation in weight loss or in decreasing body fat. Overall, the likely effect, if there is one, is small. Adolescents however, should be advised that milk drinking can be an important part of good health and will not make them gain unwanted weight. For those who are used to drinking whole milk, a gradual decrease to low-fat or to skim milk (0.5% fat) is an easily obtainable goal and can go far towards demonstrating that milk is not a high-fat or high calorie–containing food. This needs to be an ongoing family discussion with parents leading the way as good role models.

Are there any harmful effects from consuming soda related to bone health?

If dairy products are good for children's bones, and they are, despite what a few antidairy advocates say, then is soda (or *pop*) bad for your bones? Now this idea generates a lot of controversy as well. In general, regular and diet sodas are not the healthiest choice for children and, sugar–containing sodas especially should only be included in their diet as a treat, if at all. One issue concerning soda and bone health is whether phosphoric acid that is present in many regular and diet sodas causes bone loss. The data on this are mixed because there are two factors involved. First, is there any direct effect of high phosphorus or high acid intake on bones? Second, what is the *displacement* effect? That is, does drinking more soda make one drink less calcium–containing beverages including milk?

Although animal studies and a few human studies show some direct effect of high phosphorus or high-acid intake on bones, the reality is that this effect is likely minimal, especially if limited to one or two daily servings of soda (Fitzpatrick and Heaney 2003). Of course, an 8-ounce serving of soda half-filled with ice is not the same as guzzling a 20-ounce bottle! This distinction is an ever-present problem for people in understanding their dietary intake of foods. Still, it is best to focus on the second issue: the displacement effect, or the problem of drinking soda all day instead of drinking milk. There is just a limit to how much liquid a person can drink in a day. The overall amount of phosphorus in one soda is relatively little; therefore, there is no need to panic about a direct effect of one soda causing a decrease in bone calcium. The long-term effect of living on sodas, power or sports drinks, energy drinks, and such is of much more concern as it relates to bone health due to the lack of key nutrients in most of these beverages.

The same thing is true of caffeine. It is true that caffeine increases urinary calcium loss, but this effect is not large in most people, including children. There are no data in adolescents suggesting a problem with limited dietary intake of caffeine, although the available data are somewhat dated (Lloyd et al. 1998). There are much more compelling reasons to avoid supercaffeinated beverages in children and adolescents than bone health. You can read more about caffeine and diet sodas in Chapter 15 "Frequently Asked Questions" at the end of the book.

What is the most calcium that should be in the diet or taken from supplements by children and adolescents?

The tolerable upper intake limit (UL) for calcium ranges from 1000 mg per day for infants in the first six months of life to 3000 mg per day for adolescents. For the most part, there is relatively little concern about *toxic* intakes of calcium in children and adolescents (Table 9.1). Few children at any age will exceed the UL, and even those who do are unlikely to develop symptoms such as kidney stones.

In the second six months of life, the UL is set at 1500 mg per day. Again, it would be difficult for a baby to exceed this amount of calcium from formulas and usual solid foods, and impossible to even come close to it on a reasonably normal diet of breast milk with solid foods. There is no particular need for calcium supplements or high calcium–containing diets in this age group, but there are also no real problems with introducing baby foods fortified with calcium.

There has been some concern about the interaction of calcium and other nutrients. The concern is that if there is too much calcium in the diet, it will block the absorption of iron and zinc and cause anemia or other health problems. Fortunately, although this effect has been shown with short-term use of calcium supplements, it does not appear to be a problem with long-term dietary calcium or even long-term use of calcium supplements. In fact, there is some evidence that increased calcium intake blocks the toxic effect of metals, including lead from the diet. This effect is also minor in most cases. The final result is that the interaction of calcium with iron is not generally a clinical concern (Ames, Gorham, and Abrams 1999).

Table 9.1 Calcium (mg): Usual Intakes from Food, 2005–2006, Compared to Tolerable Upper Intake Levels

Gender and Age	Percentiles of Usual Intake							Upper Limit* (mg/day)
	5	10	25	50	75	90	95	
Males and females								
1 to 3 years old	494	576	728	923	1143	1364	1503	2500
4 to 8 years old	529	607	748	930	1135	1340	1467	2500
Males								
9 to 13 years old	611	688	828	1004	1211	1416	1545	3000
14 to 18 years old	565	675	893	1191	1561	1943	2197	3000
Females								
9 to 13 years old	529	603	740	921	1131	1340	1472	3000
14 to 18 years old	404	481	622	810	1044	1288	1453	3000

Source: NHANES 2005–2006, "What We Eat in America," Washington, DC: U.S. Department of Agriculture, Agricultural Research Service.

Note: Excludes breast-fed children and lactating and pregnant females.

* Institute of Medicine, 2011, *Dietary Reference Intakes for Calcium and Vitamin D*, Washington, DC: National Academy Press.

How do food companies decide what foods to fortify with calcium and bone-related nutrients? How do they decide how much to add?

Every company has its own process for making these decisions. The decisions for any fortification are based on a variety of factors we will consider below.

1. The technical side of fortifying foods

Adding high amounts of many forms of iron to food will affect the food's taste, making it have a bitter and metallic taste that is well accepted. This is not something food manufacturers are usually hoping for or willing to accept in their product. Furthermore, there may be either problems or even advantages to combining fortificants that are important. Calcium may often be added as the calcium phosphate form combining both calcium and phosphorus. Interestingly, some of these minerals may also have a preservative effect and this can be one aspect of choosing how much to add. It takes some genuine expertise in food sciences to properly fortify foods, and, therefore, not all fortified foods are of equal quality.

2. The cost of the fortificant

Now, in general, the vitamins and minerals added to foods and beverages are not very expensive to add. They are not free of charge either though, and some forms of minerals and vitamins are more expensive to add than others. Vitamin D is inexpensive but calcium may add some cost to the product. These cost considerations become very important, especially when companies are designing fortified foods for use in developing countries where even a small increase in cost may be critical in the sales and marketing of the product.

3. The target population for the product, especially if there are age-group related regulatory rules involved in the fortification

Companies marketing products for small children have to be aware of the target for the product. The companies who make these foods have to look at the dietary recommendations for babies and toddlers when deciding how much to fortify and what to add. Iron, zinc and calcium are key fortificants in baby foods because infants' diets may be lacking in these nutrients if they are not receiving a wide variety of foods.

4. Marketing of the products

Companies want to make a product that has high value and often want to add fortificants such as calcium that people will pay extra to obtain. This is called *value added* product marketing and is very important. We are all subject to this type of marketing and there are definite *buzz words* that get our attention. These include *negative* ones (*no trans fat*) and positive ones (*with antioxidants*). The people who market foods and beverages are very well aware of all the attention given to calcium and vitamin D in the media. Thus, a lot more vitamin D-fortified foods are being marketed and will be lining the shelves of your grocery store soon, with more to come. Even large fast food chains are catching on to this trend and adding calcium and vitamin D to their products.

In 2008, $2 billion was spent on marketing foods and beverages to children and adolescents. Even though the Federal Trade Commission and groups such as the U.S. Children's Food and Beverage Advertising Initiative have recommended against direct advertising of unhealthy products to children, this is voluntary, and the decisions about what constitutes an unhealthy product is left up to the manufacturer. As such, without federal interventions we expect for advertising to children to continue to grow exponentially. The recent introduction of *advergames*, which are online computer games used to market products to children, is a new media tool that can positively or negatively affect a child's food choices depending on the product being marketed.

5. Safety concerns

This is a complex issue and also related to the target population and marketing. Again, an easy example to consider is iron. A company marketing a sugar-filled iron-fortified beverage would need to be concerned if they added so much iron that a small child who drank 3 or 4 servings in a day would get a toxic iron dose. For calcium and vitamin D this is less of a concern because of wider safety margins built into the Dietary Reference Intakes (DRIs), but it is still an issue to evaluate.

6. Label claims

There are very specific rules about what you can claim on a food label, including what nutrients you can or cannot list. But the rules about other nutrition messages on the packaging are not as specific. This gives manufacturers a lot of wiggle room, and the wording of these claims plays a big role in food fortification decisions. These nutrition messages are commonly referred to as *front of package* label claims, but they could appear anywhere on the package.

There are strict Food and Drug Administration (FDA) rules about what manufacturers can say on the front of a package for certain claims. For example, the phrases *healthy, plus vitamins, excellent (or good) source of ... calcium, vitamin D (or any other vitamin or mineral), no added sugar,* and *50% less sugar* are not allowed on products intended for children under 2 years of age because appropriate dietary levels have not been established for children in this age range. A common possible violation is when the front panel shows that the product has *no trans fat,* but it does not have a disclosure statement to alert consumers that the product has significant levels of *saturated fat* and *total fat* (if it does). Another claim that is not allowed by the FDA is *excellent (or good) source of Omega-3+,* which has not been approved for use on food products.

So let us talk about what food companies are allowed to put on the front of the package that would help consumers make better choices. Over the past several years, front of package labeling has grown rampantly out of control with food manufacturers designing their own icons for nutrition messages, often in a light that made their products appear favorable and healthy. A common concept was *better for you* in which food

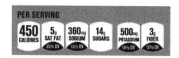

Figure 9.3 Front of package Nutrition Key icon system developed by the Grocery Manufacturers of America and the Food Marketing Institute. This is one of several ideas for helping consumers evaluate food content.

manufacturers fortified foods such as sugary cereals with vitamin D in order to promote this hot topic nutrient, but their product was still not really a nutrient rich food. Junk food fortified with extra vitamins and minerals is still basically junk food.

A report by the Institute of Medicine (IOM) in October 2010 stated that the primary purpose of any front of package labeling should be to "help consumers identify and select foods based on nutrients most strongly linked to public health concerns for Americans" (http://www.iom. edu/Reports/2010/Examination-of-Front-of-Package-Nutrition-Rating-Systems-and-Symbols-Phase-1-Report.aspx). In fact, they stated that food companies should limit front of package labeling to calories, serving size, saturated fat, trans fat, and sodium. These are nutrients most integrally involved in diseases that hit home to many Americans: obesity, cardiovascular disease, and diabetes. The IOM panel is currently in its final phase of its evaluation of front of package labeling during which they will assess which icons are most effective to communicate nutrition messages to consumers and develop a standardized icon system for all food manufacturers to use (scheduled to be released in Fall 2011).

Before the IOM panel could complete its mission, the Grocery Manufacturers Association and the Food Marketing Institute launched their own new icon system: Nutrition Keys (Figure 9.3). This voluntary approach lists calories per serving along with the amount and percentage of the Daily Value (%DV) for saturated fat, sodium, and sugars. Companies will also be allowed to list, at their discretion, two featured nutrients to encourage: potassium, fiber, protein, vitamin A, vitamin C, vitamin D, calcium, and iron. These optional nutrients can only be included if the product has at least 10% of the Daily Value for that nutrient. There are concerns that this icon system may be confusing to consumers by having too much information and that the concept of the Daily Value is still misunderstood by most of the public. A high %DV is considered unhealthy (or *bad*) for the mandatory nutrients of saturated fat, sodium, and sugars, but its considered healthy (or *good*) for the optional nutrients. And there still remains the possibility that food companies would fortify generally unhealthy foods with nutrients in order to make a front of package label claim that may mislead a consumer into thinking it is an overall healthy food.

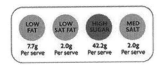

Figure 9.4 Front of package Traffic Light icons developed in Great Britain. One of several ideas being considered for evaluating food content in the United States.

One reason why the Grocery Manufacturers Association and the Food Marketing Institute have designed their own icon system definitely has to do with the upcoming IOM report. They are certainly hoping that they can persuade consumers into using their system before a new one is mandated. They are also likely trying to steer the industry away from another proposed icon system for label claims. For example, they may wish to avoid adopting the traffic light system that was previously used in Great Britain but then abandoned after criticism by the food industry. This system assigned a color code based on nutrient content: green for nutrients you should eat often, yellow for nutrients you should eat in moderation, and red for nutrients you should avoid or limit greatly (Figure 9.4). Believe us, no food company is eager to have their label covered in red warnings. Yet, what we have seen is that when the public demands and has governmental support for changes, these can happen quickly in the food supply. Just look at trans fat. As more research came out about the poor health outcomes associated with trans fat, more and more consumers demanded products that did not contain these types of fats, and food companies obliged by modifying their recipes.

Just as there is no perfect food label, there will not be a perfect front of package label. But any improvement to the current labels will be a benefit to consumers. We look forward to reading the IOM's report and hope that a new front of package label system will help consumers identify and choose healthy foods.

7. National food policies

Another interesting example of the complexity of issues with fortification is vitamin D fortification of bread. Currently, food companies are seeking to add more vitamin D to many of their products since this is a hot topic in the community, and the IOM report reflects higher requirements than previous guidelines (IOM 2011). If you want to buy a loaf of bread with extra vitamin D added to it, you are going to have to get white-wheat bread instead of 100% whole wheat bread. You would think that 100% whole wheat bread is the best and the healthiest for you. And depending on the nutrient you want to get, it might be. White-wheat bread is not just wheat bread that has been altered. It is actually a different type of albino grain that has a white color. Because there are strict rules on what can be added to 100% wheat bread, food companies cannot currently actually add any vitamin D to those products. They can however offer alternate choices through white-wheat bread. Whether the consumer realizes it or not, national food policies affect everyone, down to everyday peanut butter and jelly (on white-wheat bread) sandwiches.

8. The X factor

The whims of *who-knows-who* seem to be a part of this as well. Sometimes, we look at foods in the marketplace and cannot determine what possessed the manufacturer to add some random assortment of vitamins and minerals to the product. We will not name names as there are a lot of examples of random vitamins added to foods and beverages that seem to make people want to buy them, even though there is no apparent basis for how they were selected, nor is there the slightest evidence that the consumer or the public at large need them. Even adding 10% of the Daily Value (40 IU) of vitamin D to a bottle of water does not impress us as being all that useful in most cases. It cannot hurt, but it would not be the best reason to choose a particular product.

References

Ames SK, Gorham BM, and Abrams SA. 1999. Effects of high compared with low calcium intake on calcium absorption and incorporation of iron by red blood cells in small children. *Am J Clin Nutr* 70:44–48. Not really much concern about this interaction when viewed from the whole diet over a period of time. It is not generally necessary to separate calcium and iron in the diet or in supplements. (Free online.)

Fitzpatrick L and Heaney RP. Got soda? 2003. *J Bone Miner Res* 18:1570–2. http://www.ajcn.org/content/84/4/936.long. An argument made that moderate ingestion of soda is not a criminal act as related to bone health. In adults, an effect was seen in women but not men. Overall, soda is not a great thing for children, but, as with many other things, excessive scare tactics unaccompanied by facts do not work well with children. Moderation and rational discussion work better. More recent research related to obesity has increased the concern about sugar-containing soft drinks for children more than the concerns specific to bone health. On the whole, sugar-containing soft drinks can best be left on the grocers' shelf, not in the kitchen or in the school soda machines. (Not free online.)

Institute of Medicine. *Dietary Reference Intakes for Calcium and vitamin D*. 2011. Washington, DC: National Academy Press. See annotation in Chapter 2 "References."

Lloyd T, Rollings NJ, Kieselhorst K, Eggli DF, and Mauger E. 1998. Dietary caffeine intake is not correlated with adolescent bone gain. *J Am Coll Nutr* 17:454–7. There are lots of good reasons not to make a teenager become a caffeine addict. But, much like soda and phosphorus, the science as we present it to adolescents should be honest, and the science as reflected in this study does not really suggest a big problem with usual caffeine intakes related to bone health. The best idea is to encourage children to budget their time and get adequate sleep so they do not think they need all the caffeine. Of course, physicians who work 30-hour shifts with a coffee shop run every 6 hours are being hypocrites when they make this recommendation! That would not describe Dr. Abrams, who works 30-hour shifts in the Neonatal Intensive Care Unit (ICU) fueled by mango smoothies. (Free online.)

chapter ten

Myths and realities of vitamin D intake in children

Sunshine and vitamin D

Undoubtedly, the most controversial issue related to vitamin D is whether one should intentionally plan to obtain a significant amount of vitamin D via sunshine exposure or via artificial ultraviolet light exposure. This debate has pitted some elements of the medical community against others and has led to a tremendous amount of confusion and outright hostility between groups of physicians. Our viewpoint, as expressed here, is largely based on the perspective of the pediatric and dermatology communities, and the fundamental concept that ensuring safety is the most important thing for parents in considering sources of vitamin D for children.

Both the American Academy of Pediatrics (AAP) (Balk 2011) and the American Academy of Dermatology (Lim et al. 2001) (http://www.aad. org/skin-care-and-safety/skin-cancer-prevention/) have expressed strong concerns about the safety of relying on sunshine exposure to provide for adequate vitamin D. Both groups recommend that diet, not ultraviolet light exposure, be the key source of vitamin D for American children.

First, let us consider this issue by looking at some of the basic concepts and the controversy. Overall, it is generally accepted that the majority of the vitamin D in our bodies is produced by solar irradiation. We know this because most people have higher serum 25(OH)D levels than what we would expect from diet alone, so sunlight exposure must be contributing substantially to the overall levels. The lowest serum 25(OH)D values are found at the end of winter and in early spring compared to summer and fall, and in the northernmost parts of the United States and Canada compared to the rest of the United States. However, seasonality of vitamin D levels occurs everywhere (Unger et al. 2010). That means, even in Texas or Brazil, serum 25(OH)D levels are lower in the end of winter than in summer.

In addition, serum 25(OH)D levels are lower in populations who have dark skin compared to those with light skin, and in groups who for social or religious reasons do not expose much of their skin to the sun. Values are also lower in individuals who regularly use sunscreen, which limits irradiance-associated vitamin D conversion. A sunscreen with a sun protection factor (SPF) of 15 blocks 95% of the UV rays that lead to the conversion of vitamin D in the body; SPF 30 blocks 98% of vitamin D conversion.

Beyond these basics, controversy comes in. The available evidence has demonstrated that substantial vitamin D formation occurs in the skin sooner than tanning or especially sunburn development occurs. That is, during the summer, a fairly short exposure to the sun without sunscreen will lead to increased vitamin D levels without burning if the exposure is stopped or sunblock applied after a short period of time. It is controversial whether sun exposure for a prolonged period of time, such that substantial tanning or burning occurs, is a risk factor for skin cancer, especially melanoma, the most dangerous type of skin cancer. Nearly all members of the dermatology community strongly believe that this relationship is true, especially for melanoma. The data to properly define the length of sun exposure time needed for an increased risk of cancer based on ethnicity, season, location, sunshine exposure due to clothing (short sleeves versus long sleeves), and even whether a person is standing or lying down are minimal. Several recent papers have begun to answer these questions, although much more information is needed (Webb et al. 2011; de Gruijl 2011).

However, although the idea of very short exposures without sunscreen sounds good, in reality it is extremely difficult to do this for infants and small children. In particular, the idea of taking an infant or small child outside in the summer heat without any sunscreen for 10 to 20 minutes, then running inside, applying sunscreen and going back out for the rest of the walk or playtime just does not seem reasonably practical. It also does not take into account skin color, weather, and the realities of taking children outside on walks or to the playground.

The risk of sunburns and excessive sun exposure, while controversial, appear to be very real. Even as this field evolves, medical caregivers are seeing an increase in melanoma and other skin cancers. Although some argue that these are not related to sun exposure, animal and other data suggest this is an important relationship. We may not have a full understanding of this relationship for many years until more research is conducted. Regardless, this does not seem to be a risk worth taking for children when there are alternative sources of vitamin D such as diet and supplements. Using sunscreen, limiting sun exposure without sunscreen, and providing vitamin D via diet or supplements is our choice and the clear choice of the AAP and most similar advisory groups.

For now, we encourage families to follow this debate, but to generally be cautious with sunshine exposure without sunscreen for children and adolescents. Speak with your pediatrician or other caregiver and make the best decisions based on the opinions of those who do not have a stake in what you decide. Do not be swayed by billboards and slogans.

Skin color and calcium and vitamin D

One issue that has recently been discussed is whether there should be different dietary requirements for either calcium or vitamin D based on race
or skin color. Related to calcium, it has been known that Asians appear to
have much lower calcium intakes than Caucasians and yet do not appear
to have a high rate of bone loss or bone demineralization. Somewhat similar findings have been seen for African-Americans. Several research studies in these groups have demonstrated a greater rate of calcium absorption
compared to Caucasians despite lower serum 25(OH)D levels. The etiology
of this difference is unknown. Data also indicate that African-Americans
have less calcium loss in the urine due to a lower rate of bone turnover
(Aloia 2008).

Furthermore, it can be difficult in our current multicultural society to
identify the ethnic and racial background of individuals. Dietary patterns
in the United States compared to diets in other countries may lead to an
increased need for calcium to account for the increased calcium lost in
the urine due to high salt diets compared to a traditional diet common in
other countries.

As noted above, decreased serum levels of 25(OH)D are seen in
African-Americans compared to Caucasians. This is undoubtedly due to
decreased dermal absorption of ultraviolet light and decreased formation
of vitamin D in the skin. Interestingly, rickets in Africa is not primarily
due to vitamin D deficiency; it is much more commonly and primarily
related to extremely low calcium intakes. The serum 25(OH)D levels in
African children with rickets are usually not very low and therapy with
calcium, sometimes but not always combined with vitamin D, leads to
resolution of the rickets.

In the United States there is less milk consumption among African-
Americans compared to other ethnic groups. Most African-Americans
are at higher latitudes than their ancestors were in equatorial areas of
Africa. Vitamin D levels can be very low in some African-Americans. The
frequency of serum 25(OH)D levels less than 12 ng/mL is 10% to 20% of
African-American infants and toddlers compared to less than 2% to 3%
of Caucasians. As noted in Chapter 3, most rickets in the United States
occurs in nonvitamin D supplemented African-Americans.

There is no evidence that vitamin D is metabolized in a different way
based on race or ethnicity. Creating separate vitamin D recommendations
for African-Americans or other ethnic groups was not deemed necessary
by the Institute of Medicine (IOM) (2011). However, recognizing the lower
serum 25(OH)D levels in African-Americans, it is important to ensure that
they have an adequate intake of vitamin D based on the Recommended
Dietary Allowance (RDA). This may lead to more emphasis on fortified foods and supplements. For certain, it is critical that breast-fed and

weaning African-American infants and toddlers receive at least 400 IU per day of vitamin D.

Providing a healthy diet including calcium is a reasonable approach for all racial and ethnic groups. We do not have enough information or rationale for establishing dietary recommendations specifically based on race or ethnicity. It is doubtful that these could be properly used and do not really make much sense from a public health perspective in the United States. That does not mean that we should be unaware of ethnic and racial differences in metabolism, just that we should be cautious about trying to overuse such information rather than focusing on good health advice for everyone.

Why don't we just megadose with all the bone-related vitamins and minerals such as vitamin D? What makes doctors and dietitians reluctant to do so?

Those who would accuse the medical profession of hiding simple vitamin cures for serious conditions often appeal to the idea that doctors benefit from diseases. The idea here is expressed in different ways. Sometimes the accusation is that physicians are being paid directly by pharmaceutical manufacturers to keep the public from knowing about vitamins as a cure for diseases. Other times, the accusation is that if diseases are decreased, then doctors will be out of a job, and, therefore, doctors want to make people have more diseases. Few of these individuals note that doctors and their families would also benefit from improvements in health care. Forgotten is that physicians have been leaders in developing and testing vaccines and other measures that are central to decreasing the disease burden on children.

Few practicing pediatricians receive a substantial income from pharmaceutical firms and new federal rules are gradually leading to a decrease in this income source for physicians and making it mandatory that such payments be publicly known. Pediatricians mostly prefer to see healthy children or manage complex medical issues, not a room full of children with influenza. That is why we so strongly support full immunization of children against this and many other illnesses. Our population is aging, and illnesses in all ages are related to natural patterns of disease. In fact, modern medicine has led to a marked increase in lifespan and improvement in health.

Pediatricians and other caregivers of children are concerned that *megadosing* of a vitamin, such as vitamin D, or a mineral, such as calcium, is neither safe nor effective. Megadosing is giving vitamins or minerals at dose levels far above what is recommended by the (RDA) and sometimes above the upper limit (UL). When conspiracy theorists decide that national panels or doctors are hiding a cure, they are often ignoring the simple lack of any evidence for that cure. Offense wins, and those with the loudest voices sometimes are heard the most. There is no evidence at all for high-dose vitamin therapy of human diseases in prevention or treatment. If there were any such evidence, we would be using it for ourselves, and for our own families.

Vitamin D toxicity

An extremely contentious issue is evaluating what intake of vitamin D can be toxic. For the most part, extremely high levels of vitamin D intake are not taken by individuals due to a desire to enhance bone health. Even the strongest supporters of taking in lots of vitamin D do not usually do so primarily related to bone health, with the possible exception of the use of high-dose vitamin D during lactation to enhance vitamin D in the mother's milk. Most individuals who support vitamin D doses far in excess of the RDA do so because of its potential benefits in nonbone health conditions (Garland et al. 2011).

The issue of a toxic dose of vitamin D has been extensively discussed both in an article several years ago (Hathcock et al. 2007) and then in the IOM report (2011). In general, the consensus is that in adults, there is little suggestion of a toxic effect of vitamin D up to 10000 IU per day intake, although large population-based studies of long-term exposure to this dose are not available. Some suggest that there is little evidence of toxicity up to 80 to 120 ng/mL of serum 25(OH)D, although this remains controversial. However, for many people, doses well in excess of 10000 IU per day would be needed to reach a serum 25(OH)D of 80 to 120 ng/mL.

The IOM (2011) committee noted some emerging evidence of toxicity at lower intake levels. They were concerned about the evidence of an increase in some harmful outcomes at both very low and very high serum 25(OH)D levels in adults. This is called a *U-shape curve* because the risk of a bad outcome is greatest at the lowest and highest ranges. At this time, the evidence for a U-shape curve related to pediatric outcomes is very limited. However, the evidence of benefits for very high doses of vitamin D for most children is also not strong.

The IOM started with the 10000 IU per day dose believed to be safe and then applied a safety factor of 2.5 and set the UL for adults at 4000 IU per day. The use of the safety factor of 2.5 was relatively arbitrary. It is typical to take the lowest clearly safe dose, or the lowest dose in which any risk was actually seen and set the UL well below that, but there is no reason for it to have been exactly 2.5. Therefore, those adults who wish to take 5000 IU per day for example are on reasonable ground. Whether it would have been okay to not include a safety factor, that is, to use a safety factor of 1.0, and derive a UL of 10000 IU per day is highly controversial. It is best if this dosing level is left as a decision between an individual and his medical caregivers with close monitoring.

With regard to children, weight-based toxicological principles were applied to decrease the UL proportionally down with age to 1000 IU per day for small infants. The adult value of 4000 IU per day was used for 9 to 18 year olds. Of all of the UL values, by far the most important number is the 1000 IU per day for infants up to 6 months of age.

The risk of vitamin D toxicity, including hypercalcemia (high blood calcium) with vomiting and kidney damage, is real in healthy small infants, and there is no reason to exceed a total dose of 1000 IU per day in this group. Using the 400 IU per day guidance of the AAP and IOM is almost always the best idea in small infants. Overdosing from diet on vitamin D is very unlikely given current fortification strategies. Particular caution should be used when giving liquid forms of vitamin D to small infants. Such liquids may be very concentrated and pose an unnecessarily high risk of toxicity if accidentally overdosed. A single dose of several thousand units of vitamin D is not likely at all to cause complications even in an infant, but long-term overdosing in small infants would be a serious health concern.

Who Should Help Guide Nutrition for Children?

Good question! It is hard to know whom to trust with all the talk shows, magazines, online articles, and news reports about nutrition that are widely available. A registered dietitian (RD) is a food and nutrition expert. RD is a legally defined term, while the word *nutritionist* is not. Therefore, anyone can describe himself as a nutritionist, regardless of education, whether he has absolutely no nutrition or science classes whatsoever or a Ph.D in nutrition. Nutritionist is a completely unregulated title. In fact some RDs also use the term *nutritionist* to describe their job, but to be an RD you must have the proper education, experience such as hands-on supervised training, and knowledge to earn that credential.

There are four main steps to becoming an RD. First, you must earn a bachelor's degree from an accredited university. Coursework typically includes food and nutrition sciences including medical nutrition therapy, foodservice systems management, business, chemistry, biochemistry, physiology, and microbiology. Second, you must complete an accredited internship of 900 hours. Third, you must pass a national exam administered by the Commission on Dietetic Registration. After that, you can celebrate. Now you have the credentials of an RD! Finally, you must stay current by completing continuing educational requirements to maintain your registration.

About half of RDs also hold advanced degrees, such as a master's degree or Ph.D. Some RDs also have additional certifications in specialized areas of practice, such as pediatric nutrition, nutrition support such as tube feedings and intravenous nutrition, and diabetes education. Most RDs work in hospitals, at nursing homes, in doctor's offices, and outpatient clinics. Dietitians can also be found teaching at universities, doing research, managing school foodservice programs, working with public health programs, or providing individualized nutrition counseling in private practices, among many other nutrition related opportunities.

Hundreds of highly specialized registered dietitians work in Neonatal Intensive Care Units (NICUs) across the country. There are currently two fellowship programs for neonatal dietitians in the United States; one in Houston, Texas, and the other in Indianapolis, Indiana. Neonatal RDs discuss each NICU patient's nutritional status with the clinical team that includes physicians, nurses, residents, fellows, medical students, and pharmacists to evaluate each infant's growth, feeding tolerance, nutritional needs, vitamin and mineral supplementation, and breast milk fortification to make sure each baby is growing appropriately.

Patients in the NICU are often born prematurely and may not be able to receive any breast milk or formula because their intestines are so immature. These babies have to be provided intravenous nutrition so that they get the calories, protein, and other nutrients that they need to grow and thrive. Neonatal RDs help to make sure that these babies are getting the right balance of nutrients. Other babies in the NICU may have respiratory or cardiac issues that limit the amount of fluid, either breast milk or formula, that the baby is allowed to have. In these situations, a neonatal RD ensures that the feedings are concentrated in a safe manner in order to provide all the nutrients that a growing baby needs. If a baby needs to go home on these specialized feedings, a neonatal RD will educate the family or caregivers on the proper way to mix the products for the baby.

Another unique specialization for dietitians is pediatric nutrition. The Commission on Dietetic Registration offers Board Certification as a Specialist in Pediatric Nutrition (CSP) for registered dietitians who have a minimum of 2,000 hours of practice experience in pediatric nutrition and pass a national exam. Certification is maintained by passing the exam every 5 years. RDs who are board certified as a CSP manage the nutrition care of infants and children with special conditions such as congenital heart disease, cystic fibrosis, diabetes (type 1 or type 2), failure to thrive, food intolerances or food allergies, inflammatory bowel disease, and weight management. Education to the family and caregiver is a critical responsibility of the RD, including education regarding g 'ls and rationale of nutrition plan considering age-specific and disease-specific nutrition issues. RDs must be fully informed about the nutrient composition of specific foods in order to promote healthy eating habits and disease management.

OTHER SOURCES OF NUTRITION INFORMATION

Other good sources of information about nutrition include your child's pediatrician and publications from governmental-based research such as the United States Department of Agriculture (USDA). It is important to look for unbiased, well-researched advice on nutrition. Remember, if something sounds too good to be true, it usually is. So do not be fooled into thinking one food is the complete cause of obesity in children, or that another single food (or nutrient) is the cure-all either.

When reviewing nutrition advice, think through these concepts:

Who wrote it? Are they specialized in this field? Do they have other publications in well-respected peer-reviewed journals?

Where did the funding for the research or advice come from? Not all private corporately funded studies are bad or dishonestly conducted and reported. Most of the time, food manufacturers or infant formula companies support funding high quality research because it is good practice, and it helps them determine if changes in their products can be beneficial as well as marketable. When looking at such studies, all reputable medical journals require the scientists who have conducted a study funded by a private company to indicate the exact role the company had in the study. The best studies are those in which the funding company works closely with a well-established scientist. Most details of the design and interpretation of the study should be determined by the scientists conducting the study, not by the company sponsoring the study. This is not always possible however, and when significant corporate involvement does occur, it is a reason to be cautious about the results, although they do not need to be disregarded.

Are the claims reasonable? Do they eliminate entire food groups or nutrients? Do they make common sense? Are the claims biologically plausible? Do they reflect a whole diet? Telling people that eating bananas is healthy is reasonable, but telling them that they should eat *only* bananas is monkey business.

References

Aloia JF. 2008. African Americans, 25-hydroxyvitamin D, and osteoporosis: A paradox. *Am J Clin Nutr* 88:545S–50S. A detailed review of the differences in racial handling of calcium and vitamin D metabolism. Note especially that African-Americans have lower vitamin D levels and fewer osteoporotic fractures. (Free online.)

Balk SJ and Council on Environmental Health; Section on Dermatology. 2011. *Pediatrics* 127:e791–817. Ultraviolet radiation equals a hazard to children and adolescents. The AAP concurs that vitamin D should come from the diet, not sunshine exposure or tanning in children. They are right. That does not mean that a few minutes of sunshine is bad for children or that kids cannot play outside. Just that this should not be the primary source of vitamin D. (Not free online.)

de Gruijl FR. 2011. Sufficient vitamin D from casual sun exposure? *Photochem Photobiol* 87:598–601. This and the paper by Webb et al. discuss the length of time needed in different seasons to achieve adequate vitamin D equivalent intakes. The data are complex and not easy to translate into simple recommendations. The most important take-home is that there is no simple way to calculate the amount of time one needs to spend outside to form vitamin D or the relative safety of that.

Garland CF, French CB, Baggerly LL, and Heaney RP. 2011. Vitamin D supplement doses and serum 25-hydroxyvitamin D in the range associated with cancer prevention. *Anticancer Res* 31:607–11. Does vitamin D prevent cancer in high doses or when relatively high (e.g., > 40–50 ng/mL serum 25(OH)D levels) are achieved in the blood? This is one of the most important questions related to vitamin D intake and sun exposure in adults. Opinions and analyses of this issue are numerous and conflicting. Our opinion, consistent with the 2011 IOM report, is that the available data do not yet demonstrate on overall benefit from vitamin D on cancer rates or mortality. Others are free to disagree, but we encourage those interested in this issue to read both sides of the story. Some studies have concerning evidence that too much vitamin D may have a negative impact on some forms of cancer. (Not free online.)

Hathcock JN, Shao A, Vieth R, and Heaney R. 2007. Risk assessment for vitamin D. *Am J Clin Nutr* 85:6–18. This is one analysis regarding the safety of high-dose vitamin D supplementation. The IOM used a different approach and these can be contrasted. It is probably true that intakes up to 10000 IU per day have limited safety risks in adults and older children, but this is far from certain. (Free online.)

Institute of Medicine. 2011. *Dietary Reference Intakes for Calcium and vitamin D.* Washington, DC: National Academy Press. See annotation in Chapter 2 "References."

Lim HW, Naylor M, Hönigsmann H, Gilchrest BA, Cooper K, Morison W, Deleo VA, and Scherschun L. 2001. American Academy of Dermatology Consensus Conference on [ultraviolet A] UVA protection of sunscreens: Summary and recommendations. Washington, DC, Feb 4, 2000. *J Am Acad Dermatol* 44:505-8. The dermatologists speak virtually as one voice and have for many years advocating against the use of tanning beds and for the use of sunscreen. Arguments on this issue are intense. (Not free online.)

Unger MD, Cuppari L, Titan SM, Magalhães MC, Sassaki AL, Dos Reis LM, Jorgetti V, and Moysés RM. 2010. Vitamin D status in a sunny country: Where has the sun gone? *Clin Nutr* 29:784–8. Vitamin D levels are seasonable everywhere in the world. Even in Brazil. Time to go visit and evaluate this issue first hand! (Not free online.)

Webb AR, Kift R, Berry JL, and Rhodes LE. 2011. The vitamin D debate: Translating controlled experiments into reality for human sun exposure times. *Photochem Photobiol* 87:741–5. A bit of an obscure reference, but the conclusion is important. It does not take much sunshine to get vitamin D. That does not really answer the question as to whether this is the best approach or not. (Not free online.)

chapter eleven

Beyond bone health
Vitamin D

We have talked a good bit about strengths and limitations of scientific evidence as related to pediatric nutrition. In this chapter, we will move back to these ideas and add more detail as we explore the relationship between vitamin D and health issues in children beyond bone health.

Vitamin D functions as a hormone that is active throughout the body. Although identified almost 100 years ago as a key factor in bone health, it has increasingly become clear that vitamin D is important for more than bones. One of the original nonbone relationships identified was with skin disease. Vitamin D and its different forms, called *analogues*, are used for patients with psoriasis with great success.

In adults, there is tremendous interest in the relationship between vitamin D status and key diseases including cancer, heart disease and diabetes, among others. This is an extremely large area of research and literally hundreds of new research studies are being published each year relative to them. In 2011, the Institute of Medicine (IOM) reviewed many of the studies that had been published at that time (IOM 2011). In performing their review, the IOM relied in substantial part on a series of evidence-based reviews, including one done specifically for the IOM panel (Chung et al. 2009) (www.ahrq.gov/downloads/pub/evidence/pdf/vitadcal/vitadcal.pdf)

The IOM concluded that the data linking nonbone health-related conditions was inadequate to be used for setting dietary guidelines for vitamin D intake. That is, they concluded that more research, especially research performed using the gold-standard controlled clinical trial method, was needed before specific intake levels of vitamin D could be recommended for the prevention or treatment of any form of cancer, heart disease, or diabetes, among other conditions.

When the IOM report was released, it was widely stated that the IOM *ignored* nonbone disease or was not allowed to consider nonclinical trial evidence. Many of these statements are incorrect and misleading. The IOM report actually goes into extensive detail about nonbone disease and vitamin D, and it discusses many noncontrolled trial studies. However, the IOM panel did not agree that these data were sufficient to make recommendations about diet. Much, but not all of the IOM's perspective was based on an evidence-based review from Chung (2009) performed for the committee mentioned above. Not agreeing with something, especially when this is based on a formal evidence-based review, is not the same as ignoring it.

With regard to pediatrics, the evidence and science related to non-bone related outcomes is negligible compared to adult medicine. There are numerous conditions of importance that may have a vitamin D connection in pediatrics, however. These include type 1 diabetes and multiple sclerosis. It will be important to follow the research carefully in the future to determine if controlled trials that are being started or are underway support a role with these and other conditions. It is unfortunate how little research funding has been devoted to these relationships. Many children with chronic illnesses might be helped by nutritional intervention but extremely little research is being conducted.

Because this is a book about bone health, and because there are so little data related to nonbone health and pediatric disease, we are not able to consider all of the current potential relationships. However, we would like to discuss two diseases in pediatrics and their current scientific base. These two conditions are influenza and autistic spectrum disorder, also known as pervasive developmental disorders (henceforth *autism*). There has been considerable discussion related to these conditions and vitamin D, and so it is worthwhile to look at them.

Vitamin D and influenza

Often times, the connection between a vitamin and a disease will have some real physiological basis. Vitamin D has key roles in the immune system (Hewison 2010) and may be important in a number of disease processes, especially viral diseases and tuberculosis. Still, the clinical evidence related to pediatric diseases is extremely limited. Vitamin D, like vitamin C, does not seem to have much effect on colds and other minor respiratory illnesses. Zinc does not do much either. Chicken soup is the therapy of choice.

The connection with influenza is noteworthy both due to the force with which it is advocated, and the fact that there is a single controlled trial that looked at vitamin D supplementation and influenza in children. This study, published in the highly respected *American Journal of Clinical Nutrition* (Urashima et al. 2010) found that taking 1200 IU per day of vitamin D decreased the rate of influenza type A significantly in a group of Japanese children compared to those who did not get the vitamin D.

This sounds incredible. A moderate dose of vitamin D cut down influenza by almost half. Is it too good to be true? Well, maybe. The study had several major flaws limiting its interpretation and the certainty that this was a real relationship. The researchers did not measure serum 25(OH)D levels in any of the children. So we do not really know how the supplements affected their serum levels of vitamin D. Next, the rate of influenza overall was not significantly changed at all. Buried in the results section of the paper was the fact that influenza type B increased in these children given vitamin D supplements. Therefore there was no statistically significant benefit overall to vitamin D supplementation in the rates of influenza. Furthermore, the analysis seemed to suggest odd relationships with daycare and other factors that were not well accounted for. These issues make us concerned that the effects of vitamin D on influenza type A found in this study would not be found in another larger study. Finally, the study was much too small to make any definitive conclusions, even if U.S. children are really the same as Japanese children in terms of their exposure to infectious agents at home, school, and daycare settings.

However, many individuals were soon appearing in the media proclaiming a vitamin D victory over influenza. Some people even suggested that we should stop immunizing children, just give them vitamin D to prevent influenza. Nothing in this research study suggested that would be appropriate.

The take-home messages here are important. First, it is true that controlled trials are invaluable. But single, small, poorly controlled and analyzed trials are not reliable for public policy. Large, properly done and repeatable studies need to follow these smaller ones, and then decisions about public policy can be appropriately made. Second, immunizations are critical to decreasing the risk of influenza and saving lives. It may someday be shown that vitamin D has a role in a strategy for decreasing influenza, but we are very far from determining that. For now, we have no strong evidence that vitamin D helps decrease the incidence of influenza. Further studies should be done in a variety of populations before we go further.

Vitamin D in children: Autism

Autism is amongst the worst conditions to affect children. Parents thrilled to have a new baby slowly wonder why his development seems a bit off, but often do not make much of what may be very subtle behaviors in the first 12 to 18 months of life. Then, gradually towards the end of the second year of life it often becomes clear that the toddler is not interacting quite the way he should.

From there, it is often a whirlwind of frustration for parents during the next 12 to 24 months as they may get a solid diagnosis, but more commonly do not. Sometimes they may be told things such as "its just a mild case of autism" or "he is just a bit slow." Ultimately, once the diagnosis is made, then parents are truly swept into an awful maelstrom of standard and alternative therapies.

Given all of this, it is not surprising that alternative medicine and nontraditional ideas about the causes and treatments for autism exist and flourish. Who would not want to believe that there is a magic nutritional cure for such a terrible condition? Who can face a child they love and not hope for a solution? Often our society searches for a villain, such as vaccine manufacturers, to explain what cannot be explained.

It is not surprising then that some people have tried to find a link between vitamin D and autism (Cannell 2010). Vitamin D affects all cells of the body, and a deficiency could in theory affect neurological behavior. However, there is not the slightest meaningful evidence linking these conditions in any way as evidenced by clinical research. A few reports have attempted to link an increase in autism among African immigrants to Minnesota with vitamin D deficiency. However, a careful analysis of these reports provides no support for such a link. In fact, much of the data seems to show no connection at all or even a reverse effect (Fernell 2010). Furthermore, there are no trials of maternal or child therapies showing any relationship between autism and vitamin D.

Although some families may choose to try their autistic child on a high-dose vitamin D supplement regimen, they should be cautious about online experts recommending extremely high doses of vitamin D far above the Upper Limit (UL). Furthermore, they should be prepared to discuss this plan to provide such doses of vitamin D with their pediatric caregiver and to discontinue the high-dose supplement if they do not see an effect or if toxic effects are observed.

We believe strongly that research should be done to look at diet and autism, including the effects of vitamin D and other dietary components such as omega-3 fatty acids. Families should not, however, hold unrealistic expectations about the likely outcomes of such interventions based on the currently available scientific evidence.

Vaccines do not cause autism and vitamin D most likely does not prevent it or ameliorate it. These are realities and form the backbone of an evaluation of the current scientific and medical knowledge. New evidence may be developed that changes this view about vitamin D, but such evidence is unlikely to be available in the near future and is extremely unlikely to demonstrate a major effect of vitamin D in the treatment or prevention or autism. We would be glad to be proven wrong on this point.

Association Is Not Causation: Two Things Can Be Related to Each Other But Not Have a Causative Relationship

There are lots of things that are related to each other but not caused by each other. For example, passport holders are less likely to have type 2 diabetes (http://boingboing.net/2011/03/08/passport-ownership-p.html). This is a completely spurious relationship and does not demonstrate a direct cause and effect relationship. Obtaining a passport will not decrease a person's insulin resistance unless they use the passport to travel to a foreign country to eat well and exercise while there. This seems relatively unlikely.

Teenagers who smoke cigarettes are more likely to not graduate from an Ivy League school than teenagers who abstain from cigarettes (and a lot of other things). To conclude that tobacco or nicotine causes lower Scholastic Aptitude Test (SAT) scores is probably a stretch. Certainly we could come up with a reason for it. We could conclude that smoking decreases brain blood flow leading to poor school testing. But the reality is that there are other covariates that affect this relationship.

Covariates are the other things related to a behavior or condition that are the real, or primary things for the relationship. In our example, we know that teenagers who smoke are more likely to come from families where an Ivy League education is less common or encouraged. Even if we can find a biological link, it is probably not the real one.

If we really wanted to answer a meaningful question, we would enroll teenagers randomly into a smoking prevention program and see if those who were enrolled were more likely to be academically successful. This too would have flaws because the subjects who completed the program might be different kinds of teenagers than those who dropped out. To help deal with that, we would need to do an *intent to treat* analysis. That is, we would have to compare those who were offered the program versus those who were not regardless of whether they fully completed the program. This too is imperfect. Furthermore, even if we found an effect, we would wonder if we had missed the real *causation*. Maybe participating in the program to stop smoking caused teens to become more engaged with the program mentors and improved their approach to school. It might be that the actual reason is not important to us. Just creating such a program might be a goal regardless of how it worked.

These types of false or uncertain cause and effect associations are especially true in nutritional sciences. So it may be with vitamin D. When we look at people who have low serum 25(OH)D levels, we see an increased risk of many common diseases. But, there are challenging covariates involved. Many illnesses lead people to spend less time outdoors, or to be overweight, or to not have a good diet. It is not surprising then that many of these conditions are associated with low serum 25(OH)D levels. Add in complex genetic factors, and it becomes even tougher to sort out the cause and effect relationships.

There are several ways to deal with this, each having substantial limitations. The first is to statistically adjust for these covariates using mathematical methods. That is, if one is concerned about the relationship between type 2 diabetes and vitamin D, then in analyzing these relationships it is important to include body weight and/or body mass index (BMI) as a covariate. This can help, but is an imperfect solution in many cases.

A second approach is to perform physiologic studies of a relationship. These are important and can take many forms. They might be studies involving cells, animals, or humans in which doses of vitamin D are given and biological endpoints (e.g., insulin levels) are measured. Such studies give important insights into physiology but do not prove relationships. Humans are neither rats, pigs, nor cell cultures, and many times these physiology experiments do not represent the human physiology well.

A third approach is to actually do a trial of vitamin D supplementation and see whether the condition of interest is decreased. Such studies are extremely expensive costing often many millions of dollars, difficult to perform, and take years to do. They are subject to flaws in design, and controversy about dosing and outcomes that can lead some to doubt the final response. They are, however, absolutely needed (Shapses and Manson 2011; Manson 2010). Controlled trials have stunned the medical and nutritional world in recent years. They have shown that estrogen is not entirely safe for postmenopausal women and that high doses of vitamin E may not be safe either, although this remains extremely controversial (http://nutrition.about.com/od/researchstudies/a/vitaminestudy.htm).

Whenever you hear that nutrients, including vitamin D, *cannot* be studied by such trials, this is not accurate. For sure we cannot try *no food* or *no vitamin* versus *food* or *vitamin*, but we can determine if supplementation above usual or recommended amounts has any benefit. Those who advocate for dosing of any nutrient well above the Recommended Dietary Allowance (RDA) should insist that such studies be done to evaluate both safety and efficacy.

References

Cannell JJ. 2010. On the aetiology of autism. Acta Paediatr 99:1128–30. E-pub May 19, 2010. Opinion, not based on evidence, even when stated repeatedly and via Web sites and e-mail, does not equal proof. Neither do small numbers of individual cases unaccompanied by any medical evaluation or documentation prove an effect such as this. However, a few people believe in this relationship passionately, so we should evaluate it further using well done and properly controlled studies. Shortcuts should not be done in evaluating this question. Studies should be started prenatally with long-term follow-up throughout early childhood. (Free online.)

Chung M, Balk EM, Brendel M, Ip S, Lau J, Lee J, Lichtenstein A, Patel K, Raman G, Tatsioni A, Terasawa T, and Trikalinos TA. 2009 *vitamin D and Calcium: A Systematic Review of Health Outcomes. Evidence Report No. 183.* (Prepared by the Tufts Evidence-based Practice Center under Contract No. HHSA 290-2007-10055-I.) AHRQ Publication No. 09-E015. Rockville, MD: Agency for Healthcare Research and Quality. This was the evidence-based review related to calcium and vitamin D done for use by the 2011 IOM panel. More about this can be found in the IOM report (http://books.nap.edu/openbook. php?record_id=13050&page=725). An alternative reference can be found searching PubMed for PMID: 20629479. (Available free online at this address: www.ahrq.gov/downloads/pub/evidence/pdf/vitadcal/vitadcal.pdf.)

Fernell E, Barnevik-Olsson M, Bågenholm G, Gillberg C, Gustafsson S, and Sääf M. 2010. Serum levels of 25-hydroxyvitamin D in mothers of Swedish and of Somali origin who have children with and without autism. *Acta Paediatr* 99:743–7. These data simply do not show any connection between vitamin D deficiency and autism. If anything, they point to no relationship at all. (Not free online.)

Hewison M. 2010. Vitamin D and the immune system: New perspectives on an old theme. *Endocrinol Metab Clin North Am* 39:365–79. There are many detailed reviews of the interaction of the immune system with vitamin D. Pick the one at your level of immunology knowledge to read. (Not free online.)

Institute of Medicine. 2011. *Dietary Reference Intakes for Calcium and vitamin D.* Washington, DC: National Academy Press. See annotation in Chapter 2 "References."

Manson JE. 2010. Vitamin D and the heart: Why we need large-scale clinical trials. *Cleve Clin J Med* 77:903–10. Great article describing the need for real clinical trials of vitamin D and the ongoing trial Dr. Manson is directing of vitamin D and omega-3s. Unfortunately, it will be several more years, perhaps about 2015–2016 before we have these results. Of note is that the trial is already being criticized due to the subjects chosen and doses. There is no perfect controlled trial, but if vitamin D has an effect on major health outcomes, and it is not seen in this study, that will be important information. If it is seen, or if seen in conjunction with omega-3s, that would potentially be a reason to reevaluate the Dietary Reference Intakes (DRIs) for vitamin D related to these outcomes. (Free online.)

Shapses SA and Manson JE. 2011. Vitamin D and prevention of cardiovascular disease and diabetes: why the evidence falls short. *JAMA* 22;305:2565–6.. More about why we just do not have enough evidence yet for these key outcomes. (Not free online.)

Urashima M, Segawa T, Okazaki M, Kurihara M, Wada Y, and Ida H. 2010. Randomized trial of vitamin D supplementation to prevent seasonal influenza A in schoolchildren. *Am J Clin Nutr* 91:1255–60. Small trial with severe limitations not the least of which is that overall influenza cases were not decreased. Suggestive of an effect, but much more evidence is needed. Immunizations are still first line of prevention in our opinion, and it is inappropriate for anyone to use this study as a reason not to get a flu shot.

chapter twelve

Putting it all together

Bone health as part of good nutrition for infants and children

It would be an understatement to say that families are getting mixed, confused, and sometimes, completely impossible to understand messages about nutrition today. Many of these messages contain information or guidance about bone health. For example, advocates of vegan diets sometimes insist that milk is bad for your bones. Advocates for low carbohydrate diets and low sugar diets often argue that children should not drink any flavored drinks or juices. Advocates for suntan booths argue that adolescents should be allowed to use these booths in order to increase their vitamin D. In contrast, other public advocacy groups have argued for banning children under age 18 from suntan booths.

So it goes endlessly. Oftentimes the bone message is caught up in part of a bigger advocacy (low versus high fat, vegetarianism, organics, breastfeeding, and so forth), and sometimes, it is part of the main message. Regardless, it is nearly impossible to sort out, and policies related to how foods are packaged and labeled make this even more difficult at times.

Fundamentally, it is possible to have a bone-healthy diet no matter what *big picture* diet you choose for yourself, your children, or your children pick for themselves. Any diet, except one that is truly nutrient deficient (e.g., as might be chosen by a young adolescent with an eating disorder), can be provided in a bone-healthy way. Furthermore, regardless of diet, other healthy practices, including exercise are essential to developing life-long strong bones.

Summary: Infants

When it comes to infants, the food of choice as a primary source of bone-related nutrients is breast milk. Breast milk contains everything a healthy term or late preterm infant needs in the first six months of life for growth and development except adequate amounts of vitamin D and maybe iron from 4 to 6 months. For babies who are not breast-fed, every infant formula sold in the United States and almost any country worldwide will have plenty of nutrients needed for health. That does not mean that infant formula is a perfect replacement for human milk. Only that when breast milk is not available for an infant, one can be certain from a bone mineral perspective that there is no risk to the infant from using any standard infant formula prepared properly based on the manufacturer's instructions. The suggestion to provide specialized formulas as a supplement for breast-fed infants is a costly one that is not evidence-based.

However, there are some issues to be cautious about. First, is the use of nonhuman milk, nonformula, feeding for infants. This includes goat's milk and other milks not specifically approved by the Food and Drug Administration (FDA) for infant feeding. Goat's milk is potentially deficient in folic acid and high in phosphorus. Animal milks other than cow's milk are not designed or approved for infant feeding unless specifically designated as such. Second is the use of high-dose vitamin D supplements. Adults can definitely take up to 4000 IU per day of vitamin D, and it is possible that up to 10000 IU per day or even more is safe. But newborn infants should not be given more than a total of 1000 IU each day, and there is no proven need for any healthy infant to get more than a 400 IU daily as a supplement. Future research might define a group of infants at higher risk for vitamin D deficiency that would benefit from more vitamin D, but for now, available data for infants in the United States and Canada do not demonstrate such a need. It is important that breast-fed infants begin their vitamin D as soon as possible, preferably in the first few weeks of life.

Older infants are in motion. They crawl, they stand, they walk, and they get infections such as virally caused diarrhea and ear infections. Through all of this, however, they do not really need much more calcium or vitamin D than smaller babies. There is a balance such that plenty of calcium is obtained from a diet of human milk or formula when supplemented with a small amount of solid foods. It is not necessary to choose a special *toddler formula* for children older than 9 months of age (see "Summary: Toddlers" following) or pick baby foods that are marketed as being high in calcium. For certain, it is not necessary to choose a *flavored* beverage for children in the second six months of life.

Summary: Toddlers

The requirement for calcium is relatively easy to achieve for most toddlers, as bone growth does not accelerate during the second year of life. The overwhelming majority of toddlers will get plenty of all of the dietary components needed for bone health from their diet if milk is a part of their diet along with some cheeses and yogurts.

Vitamin D requirements increase to a Recommended Dietary Allowance (RDA) of 600 IU per day during the second year of life. This would be the amount in 1.5 liters of milk, if that were the only source of vitamin D. Clearly, that is not appropriate and would be a risk for over-weight and iron deficiency. Therefore, to reach 600 IU per day requires some additional dietary creativity, or the use of a liquid vitamin supplement. One could also consider that although the RDA is 600 IU per day, this is probably not an absolute need for all toddlers. Coming close via diet, as long as the intake is over 400 IU per day is probably adequate. Children who are not given any form of milk or specialized formulas in the second year of life would need calcium and vitamin D supplements in most cases.

Whether alternative milk sources, including calcium and vitamin D-fortified soy, almond, and other beverages provide enough bioavailable calcium as an alternative in this situation is unknown. It is likely that this is the case, although the bioavailability may be somewhat below that of human milk or cow's milk. More research is needed regarding the bioavailability of minerals from these types of milks, especially in small children. Unfortunately, this is not easy to do as many specialized milks contain multiple forms of calcium, for example, making testing of bio-availability very difficult or nearly impossible.

Notably, research has shown that exercise is already important in bone health, even at this early age. Of course, it is hard to prevent a healthy toddler from exercising, especially their temper!

Summary: Early school-age children (ages 4–8)

This is an inadequately studied age group. On the one hand, bone growth does not accelerate in the prepubertal child. The overall rate at which calcium goes into the skeleton is only slightly higher than in the smaller child. However, several studies have suggested a substantial effect whereby more calcium in the diet of children shortly before the pubertal growth spurt enhances bone growth. Therefore, it is reasonable to increase emphasis on maintaining a good calcium intake of about 1000 mg per day in the prepubertal child.

It is important in this age group to focus on the development and maintenance of overall good dietary habits. Children in this age group are influenced by the diets of their parents, their older siblings, and their friends. So, overall good diet probably trumps specific emphasis on calcium and vitamin D. Specifically, high calorie, high-sugar cereals should not be chosen for children just because they are vitamin D fortified! When everyone in the family is drinking milk, it is likely that the children in this age group will do so too. Skim milk, 0.5%, or at most 1% milk should usually be the standard in this age group and older children and adults.

With regard to meeting the 600 IU per day RDA of vitamin D, again this is a challenge for most children. Consideration of a small multivitamin supplement should be made (see Chapter 5 "Picking a Multivitamin").

If this is not chosen, then 3 dairy servings and some effort to include high vitamin D–containing foods will be needed to come reasonably close to the 600 IU per day. Again, as with younger children, it is not necessarily crucial to ingest 600 IU every day,

Summary: Adolescents

A large part of bone growth and mineralization occurs during adolescence. It is important to note that *adolescence* in bone terms means from about the beginning of puberty until, for girls, about 2 to 3 years after their first menstrual period (called *menarche*), and for boys until about ages 16 to 18 years. So, the start time is age 9 to 10 in general, especially for girls. During this time, the dietary requirement for calcium goes up. The RDA is 1300 mg per day, although it is likely that intakes of 800 to 1100 mg per day are typically needed as a minimum to support bone mineralization. Regardless, many adolescents fall well below any of these targets and as many as one-third of girls are far below recommended intakes taking in less than 500 to 600 mg per day of calcium from diet or supplements. The effects of these very low intakes may be substantial in terms of achieving peak bone mass.

Reaching these intake goals requires paying considerable attention both to diet and attitudes towards diet. If teenage girls believe, very incorrectly, that milk drinking will make them become overweight, and decrease their dairy intake, while increasing their diet soda intake, then that is a real problem for parents to address. As with many things, children in this age group continue to model their behaviors, in part, based on what they see their parents do. If parents are drinking soda (or alcohol) rather than milk at key meals, then adolescents may do so as well.

Adolescence is also a time to ensure that children have plenty of vitamin D and other vitamins and minerals, including iron, in their diet. It is less crucial to focus on a single nutrient, even vitamin D, than a comprehensive healthy diet. The RDA of 600 IU per day will be challenging, but possible to reach from diet alone. Diet, including dairy products and possibly a small supplement should be enough to provide vitamin D for most adolescents.

Summary: Maternal nutrition

Most pregnant and lactating women will be adequately served by a diet that has the RDA intake levels of calcium and vitamin D. This is 600 IU per day of vitamin D and 1000 mg per day of calcium. Adolescents who are pregnant or lactating should receive 1300 mg per day of calcium. In general, this amount can be achieved using either a good, dairy–containing diet with a prenatal supplement vitamin, or by taking small extra supplements of calcium and vitamin D along with a prenatal supplement.

There are ongoing studies about high-dose vitamin D supplements (4000 to 6000+ IU per day) in both maintaining a healthy pregnancy and in providing enough calcium in milk for babies. At the present time, we do not advocate these high doses for routine use, but we recognize that some women may choose to take these higher doses and, overall, they are probably safe. More research is needed in this area however. Additionally, pregnant and lactating women whose natural intake of calcium is low would probably benefit from taking some supplemental calcium, usually not more than 500 mg of calcium once or twice daily to be sure of being at or slightly above the RDA.

Supplement containing pills providing more than 1000 mg per day of calcium are probably not beneficial during pregnancy or lactation and should be avoided. An exception might be those women at high risk for hypertensive disorders of pregnancy who should discuss the best approach to calcium supplementation with their primary caregivers.

From a maternal health perspective, being sure that the mother is overall in the best nutritional shape possible, such as having a body mass index that is as close to possible as ideal and having a good overall diet with adequate iron is more important than focusing on bone health. Ensuring plenty of folic acid in the diet or by supplement before conceiving and preventing and treating anemia are also important.

Keep an eye out for ongoing research and recommendations related to maternal bone health and calcium and vitamin D. This remains an area with many opinions, some research, and virtually no consensus.

Growth Curves

How do we determine growth in children? Pediatricians go to the growth charts from the Center for Disease Control (CDC) and pick pink for girls and blue for boys. We are all familiar with the lines on these growth curves that are used to plot growth during childhood. But, where did these curves come from? What is the basis for them? Should different growth curves be used based on a child's race, ethnicity, or the height of her mother and father? What if our child is breast-fed compared to formula-fed? What about a child with a genetic problem such as Down syndrome?

Let's briefly consider some of these issues. First, the curves that are most widely used in the United States come from the CDC. Almost everyone reading this in the United States and many other countries, was, as a child, plotted on curves that were developed many decades ago based primarily on healthy, Caucasian, formula-fed babies in the United States.

A number of years ago, a group of investigators began to wonder if this was the right dataset to use. Studies in the 1980s and 90s were showing that breast-fed infants had different growth patterns than formula-fed infants (Dewey 1998). Specifically, breast-fed infants grew slightly faster in weight initially and then slowed down in weight growth by about 3 months of age compared to formula-fed babies. This resulted in growth curves for exclusively breast-fed infants that made it look like they were not growing adequately as they were decreasing percentiles on the growth curves after about 2 to 3 months of age. Publications in that era advised pediatricians and others of this issue and reminded them that breast-fed infants who were decreasing percentiles might not actually be having any problems with growth. However, curves often won out and many a mother was advised to add other foods or switch to formula.

This problem was especially severe for infants who were born small for dates, also called, *small for gestational age*, (SGA) or premature. Such infants might have started at about the 5th percentile on the curve if they were breast-fed. They would subsequently *fall off* the graph and sometimes mothers were told to stop breast-feeding them due to presumed growth failure. Length growth usually did not fall off the curve, but few people seriously focus on length growth in evaluating overall growth of most infants and small children.

The solution to this problem was the development of new growth curves. These curves were developed by a global team of experts based on infants and children from throughout the world. A major effort and remarkable in scope, it is described from the World Health Organization (WHO) Web site as follows:

> The WHO Multicentre Growth Reference Study (MGRS) was undertaken between 1997 and 2003 to generate new growth curves for assessing the growth and development of infants and young children around the world. The MGRS collected primary growth data and related information from approximately 8500 children from widely different ethnic backgrounds and cultural settings (Brazil, Ghana, India, Norway, Oman and the USA). The new growth curves are expected to provide a single international standard that represents the best description of physiological growth for all children from birth to five years of age and to establish the breastfed infant as the normative

> model for growth and development. (Accessed August 2011
> *http://www.who.int/childgrowth/mgrs/en/*).
>
> Infants were enrolled and followed who were fed based on
> WHO guidelines. That is, infants followed in the study were
> primarily breast-fed in early life. They were not subject to
> severe economic limitations in obtaining food later in infancy,
> even in the relatively low resource countries in which parts of
> the study were conducted.

What did this process of developing new growth curves show? Well, first, it showed that there was very little difference in the growth rates of infants throughout the world who were appropriately fed. Despite differences in race and ethnicity, when fed based on what we believe to be the best practices in infant and early childhood nutrition, infants and small children in different societies grow at about the same rate.

Second, it showed, as expected, that there were substantial differences between the older curves used by the CDC and the data from this study. In brief, as seen in the small earlier studies, breast-fed babies grew a bit faster initially than the ones in the older curves, but then their growth, especially their weight growth slowed down. After 24 months of age, there was very little difference between the newer curves from the WHO and the older CDC curves (Grummer-Strawn et al. 2010).

In deciding how to proceed, the CDC has currently chosen to recommend using the new WHO standard for all infants up to 24 months of age. They recommend continuing to use the older curves for children over 24 months of age, primarily due to the fact that there are few differences in the curves and the older curves go throughout childhood and adolescence whereas the new WHO curves stop at age 5 years. Finally, they recommended using the new lower lines on the growth curves, set at the 3rd and 97th percentile (two standard deviations above or below average) compared to the commonly used 5th and 95th percentiles used previously. Visit http://www.cdc.gov/mmwr/preview/mmwrhtml/rr5909a1.htm and http://www.cdc.gov/growthcharts/.

Returning to the issue of overall growth, it is important for parents to remember that weight growth is only one part of determining if a child is growing adequately. Length and head circumference are very important, perhaps more important than weight when undernutrition is a serious concern in an individual child. Head growth is not a perfect marker for neurological outcome, but they are related. A high-risk infant whose head is not growing well is one whose nutrition should be considered carefully and an evaluation for inadequate nutrition undertaken. Length in infants up to 2 years of age is assessed with the child lying down, using a length board, and must be performed by two people to be accurate. Mostly, parents of infants like to plot the length to brag about how big their baby has gotten. But, it is important in some cases, such as formerly very premature or very low birth weight infants, to obtain and plot an accurate length.

More thorough assessment of growth may also involve measurement of body composition including the measurement of the mid-upper arm circumference, and, where available skin-fold thicknesses. The use and misuse of these values is an important topic especially in global nutrition research and policy.

References

Dewey KG. 1998. Growth characteristics of breast-fed compared to formula-fed infants. *Biol Neonate* 74:94–105. One of several review papers that preceded the new WHO growth curves discussing the different growth characteristics of infants who are breast-fed versus those who are formula-fed. Remember always that breast-fed is the normal growth pattern. (Not free online)

Grummer-Strawn LM, Reinold C, Krebs NF, and Centers for Disease Control and Prevention (CDC). 2010. Use of World Health Organization and CDC growth charts for children aged 0–59 months in the United States. *MMWR Recomm Rep.* September 10;59(RR-9):1–15. After all, your tax dollars support this work! A great read about the new WHO growth curves. Key information: "Clinicians should be aware that fewer U.S. children will be identified as underweight using the WHO charts, slower growth among breastfed infants during ages 3 to 18 months is normal, and gaining weight more rapidly than is indicated on the WHO charts might signal early signs of overweight." (Free online.)

chapter thirteen

Unanswered questions
How do we conduct and publicize good nutritional research?

One theme that we have tried to focus on is our belief that the scientific information with which we make very important dietary decisions regarding infants, children, and adolescents is woefully inadequate. Furthermore, the information sources we have available to us regarding the scientific evidence are often inaccurate and distorted. Very frequently, there is confusion between two things being associated with each other and those two things being causally related. Despite this obvious reality, every day there are numerous articles, widely quoted, which make just that incorrect leap and link two things without much evidence of a cause and effect relationship between them.

In terms of both the bone health and the nutrients of importance including calcium, phosphorus, magnesium, zinc, vitamin D, and others, there are very few well-performed research studies that truly tell us if taking supplements, especially those leading to total intakes above the Recommended Dietary Allowance (RDA), makes a long-term difference in the health of children. It is crucial that these studies be performed. Osteoporosis is a serious, widespread, and debilitating disease. Understanding how to prevent it beginning in childhood is crucial. Yet, we have virtually no research telling us the answers to this that track children over a long period of time.

For medications, we demand to have them tried in what are called *placebo-controlled trials*. Sometimes the comparison is against nothing that is thought to have any biological activity (*placebo*) and sometimes against the current therapy. For nutrition, such studies are not commonly done, and when done, often give very different answers than were expected. Placebo controlled trials showed that selenium and vitamin E were not beneficial in preventing prostate cancer (Lippman et al. 2009), that calcium did not prevent preterm delivery in the United States, and, in a very famous example, that estrogen therapy had serious risks for postmenopausal women. All of these findings were in direct contrast to what was expected based on nonrandomized trials.

We must demand a high standard for nutritional research in children. There are those who claim we cannot do this, because nutrients cannot be left out of a diet. This is true but incomplete in explaining the situation. We cannot give a child a diet with no calcium and see what happens to them. However, we can compare those who take average amounts of calcium to those who take high-dose supplements and have total intakes well above the RDA. This is what is commonly done in many studies. However, such studies are neither inexpensive nor fast. We need to be patient and demand good research before jumping to conclusions.

One of the most important areas for research is in determining what truly is an *optimal* level of serum 25(OH)D at any age, and whether there are real health benefits of testing individuals for serum 25(OH)D or high-dose vitamin and mineral supplements. Honestly, our history of demanding certain blood testing and dietary intake levels (e.g., cholesterol below 200 mg/dL and dietary fat below 30%) has not been one of great success.

In pediatrics, highly targeted testing is likely the way to go for both serum 25(OH)D testing and even for bone mineral density testing by Dual-Energy X-ray Absorptiometry (DXA). It seems very unlikely based on the present evidence that either of these tests offers much as routine testing for healthy children at any age. Whether it offers anything for those with dark skin, those who are obese, or even those with many chronic illnesses needs research, and this should be done immediately. What it means in terms of bone health to be of high-risk racially or ethnically, or to have a chronic illness is poorly defined. This research needs to be prospective, properly controlled for environmental, genetic factors, and diet, and based on meaningful biological outcomes.

It can be helpful in understanding why we lack such important research to understand some details of how such research is designed and carried out. Everyone, including us, demands high quality research. Few, however, are familiar with all of the challenges in doing such research. We have spent decades in this area, and conducted and published dozens of studies on nutrition in children, and this is a chance to provide some information on clinical research in this area. Virtually nothing is written in this area that is not designed for experts. Therefore, here is a little sample of a typical study design, with commentary on what the issues and costs involved in the research might be. This example is designed to provide some insight into the challenges of conducting clinical research on children, not to actually answer the question in our example.

Let's begin to design a study to answer the question, "What are the effects of a low vitamin D status on migraines in children?" This sounds like a really easy question to answer. Now, keep in mind that we are not neurologists and not experts in migraines, but the research approaches we are proposing here are not specifically dependent on the detailed physiology of migraines. There are those who believe that migraines are related to vitamin D deficiency but there are no clinical trials in pediatrics to answer the question. So, it should be easy; give some children vitamin D and see if their migraines go away! Not so fast, however. There are many things to consider in making such a *simple* study a reality.

The first thing we would need would be a study objective and a primary study hypothesis. The objective might be, "To determine if children who suffer recurrent headaches benefit from vitamin D supplementation." The hypothesis related to this objective might be, "We hypothesize that children who have serum 25(OH)D levels less than 30 ng/mL will have a significant decrease in migraines if given enough vitamin D to obtain a serum level of at least 40 ng/mL." Alternately, we could consider a study hypothesis such as, "We hypothesize that a daily dose of 2000 IU per day of vitamin D will significantly decrease the frequency of migraines." These are vastly different hypotheses and would require very different study designs to evaluate.

Now, all of this sounds simple but we already have created far more questions about the study design than we have answered. Therefore, here are some of the questions we need to consider immediately. This is just a minimal list of the challenges in conducting such a research study. We note that the questions below are a real aspect of our process of setting up and conducting a study. They are not theoretical concerns but real issues in pediatric research.

1. What age group do we want to study? Has this question already been studied in adults? If we want to study children, then how do we ensure that the study is safe and has benefits for the children who participate? If there are no benefits to the children who participate, how do we make this clear in the consent process in which they and their parents will participate? Are we certain that children will not be harmed by any procedure or medication that is part of the study?

2. Is it ethical to do a placebo-controlled trial for this type of question? This is a very challenging issue and probably depends on the usual vitamin D status of the population, as well as one's own view of what a low status is. Also, what is meant by *placebo* in this study? Would you compare 2000 IU daily vitamin D supplementation versus no supplementation, for example, or would you compare 2000 IU per day versus the RDA of 600 IU per day? Would you encourage sunshine exposure? Would you limit it? How would you assess it?

3. Whom would you include and exclude in your trial? Would you do a screening serum 25(OH)D and decide whether or not to include someone according to their baseline serum 25(OH)D? If so, you will need consent and Institutional Review Board (IRB) ethics committee approval just for that, not to mention funding for it. Would it be

ethical to include a subject with a serum 25(OH)D of 5 ng/mL? What about one with 60 ng/mL? What about one who was already taking 2000 IU per day of vitamin D? If the serum 25(OH)D level was less than 12 ng/mL are you obligated to refer the child to a physician for evaluation and therapy? How would you assess the potential subject's medical history to be sure they would qualify?

4. Once you have decided on all of this, what you then must do is begin to think about study design issues. One of the first would be to decide what you would consider to be the definition of a child with *migraines* and who would have had to make this diagnosis. Lots of children have headaches, but only some of these are classified as migraines. Most headaches are not migraines, and making a wrong classification would likely ruin your study. Would you require a pediatric neurologist to make the diagnosis? How often would you require that the children have migraines? Some migraines are related to menstrual cycles so you will need information about this and about contraception use. The IRB may ask you to determine if the subject is pregnant before allowing them to enroll. How will you handle these issues? If you were studying adolescents, it would be best to know what their pubertal development was. However, optimally, this requires an external examination by a physician or nurse of their genitalia to determine the level of pubertal development based on an established scale called the *Tanner Score*. Will this be permitted by the IRB? Will the subjects and their parents agree to this?

5. Where are you going to find these children? Are you going to advertise to the public for your research? Public ads like this can be very expensive. Are you going to send out letters to pediatricians and pediatric neurologists that usually have a very low return rate? Are you going to work from clinics for the underserved?

6. What type of an effect would you be looking to find? Would you be happy if the treatment with high-dose vitamin D decreased migraines by 50%? 20%? Would you be happy if an effect occurred in one-third of the subjects? Are you trying to find a *statistical effect* or a biologically important effect? How would you decide this?

7. Do you care about the frequency and severity of migraines or just the frequency? It seems reasonable that if there is a vitamin D effect, that some individuals might still get migraines, just not as bad or as long-lasting. How would you account for this in your study design? How often do you plan to ask the subjects about their migraines?

8. Studies in children are challenging when the outcome is pain or other physical symptoms. A *pain diary* might be typical but you would need older children (usually over age 12 or so) for this. That would probably be acceptable for this study, but if the outcome you

were looking at was something like influenza or respiratory illness, you would want to also study young children and this type of information can be hard to obtain.

9. Almost any adolescents or adults with migraines serious enough to be involved in your study will also be receiving other therapies. These include basic things like resting, low-light, and basic pain medicine such as ibuprofen. It also frequently includes prescription-only medications such as Sumatriptan (Imitrex) and a range of similar medications. Which of these would you permit in your study? How would you make such decisions?

10. How do you account for other *covariates* including other illnesses the subjects might have, pubertal development, ethnicity, and gender? In general, you want to balance these factors between the therapy and placebo; but the more of these factors that are important, the more difficult it is, the more subjects you need, and, of course, the more expensive the study. For example, if you randomize subjects based only on gender to get high or low doses of vitamin D, then you may have an imbalance of those who have or have not reached menarche. If you randomize by multiple factors, then each group becomes smaller. There are ways to deal with this in the statistical analysis, but each factor adds a challenge to ensuring that the placebo and the intervention are balanced in group size and characteristics.

Now, suppose we take a stab at answering a few of the key questions above so we can move forward. Let's study 14 to 18 year olds who have been diagnosed by a pediatrician or pediatric neurologist with classic migraines and have at least one attack a month. We would like to find a 25% reduction in the frequency of these attacks over a year as our primary outcome; and, as a secondary outcome, find a decrease of 20% in the number of days of school or work that are missed due to headaches. We will start the study at any time of the year, and continue it for a whole year in each child in order to account for some of the effects of season of the year on vitamin D levels. We will compare a supplement of 400 IU per day to a supplement of 2000 IU per day in a double-blind controlled trial.

We will not prescreen for vitamin D levels as this is too cumbersome to do, but will exclude anyone who routinely takes a pill supplement with more than 400 IU per day of vitamin D. We will also exclude anyone with any other severe health problem, but include children in the study who have an attention deficit disorder. We will also include girls who are receiving hormonal pills for any reason. We will recruit by sending flyers to every pediatrician in the city and by offering subjects a small amount of money for participating, perhaps $50. This will be carefully considered by the ethics committee due to concerns about coercion of children to participate in research by being paid. Some IRBs might not permit any payment at all which will make recruitment much more difficult. After all, vitamin D is not something that a family can only get by participating in this study. If they hear about the study, and that there is a 50% chance of getting placebo, a family could reasonably just decide to go buy some vitamin D and refuse to participate. We will not do physical exams but will have a questionnaire assessing issues related to pubertal development and menstrual history. We will need to do a urine pregnancy screen on all of the females as the IRB demands it. We will hope and pray that none of these screens are positive and we have to deal with that.

How many study subjects would it take to answer this question? Well, it depends on the frequency of migraines one expects in this population and the decrease you expect to find with the vitamin D therapy. There are specialized statistical programs to evaluate how many subjects are needed to have at least an 80% or 90% chance of finding the effect you are looking for. This is often called the *study power*.

We will not attempt to do the calculations for this study here, but it would not be unusual for this type of research to need at least 100 subjects in both the treatment and placebo arm to find a decrease in the symptoms that would be expected to be meaningful. For some outcomes, many more than 100 subjects would be needed, and for a few outcomes, one could find an effect with fewer subjects. Mostly, however, several hundred subjects at least are needed for clinical trials of this sort.

Now, all of this sounds great but we need to figure out how much this study would cost and who would pay for it. It is difficult to put cost estimates on this study without a clearer concept of how the study would be done, but there is little doubt that such a study would cost several hundred thousand dollars, quite possibly a million dollars or more. This would include the need for a study coordinator, dietitian, principal scientist, statistician, and others to give their time and expertise. These individuals do not and should not work for free. A lab testing arrangement would be needed as well as a research pharmacy to prepare and *blind* the placebo and therapy doses of vitamin D. Assistants would be needed to collect the data on migraines, enter it into computer programs, and interpret the results.

The only realistic primary source of funding for this study would by the National Institutes of Health (NIH) most likely via the R01 (individual research) mechanism. Currently less than 20% of such grants are funded and the chance of this type of study being funded is not terribly high. Unfortunately, there is no real chance of any corporate funding and many would not wish to use corporate funding for this type of research. Why would a company fund this since there is no proprietary medication involved?

Even if funded, the time it takes to get such a grant, and conduct and interpret a 1-year vitamin D intervention study is at least 4 years, or more likely, 5 years or more. This type of research does not happen quickly.

Overall, it is much, much easier to propose to study the effects of calcium, vitamin D, or any such intervention than it is to actually conduct the study. That does not mean such studies should not be done, but it does mean that we cannot expect quick or easy research answers to these questions.

How do we publicize the study results once we are done?

Medical schools, hospitals, and the like all have great publicity departments these days. We have a lot of respect for these departments. After all, if we want to tell the world what we know, then we need public relations professionals to help us get the message out. However, sometimes the research message gets distorted and a negative turns into a positive. We have discussed this earlier in the book related to calcium and bone health in children, but want to consider it more.

First, let's consider what it means to have a significant positive finding in a scientific study. In general, this is interpreted in the scientific and medical literature as having a $p < 0.05$ that the difference found between groups was just due to chance. What does this mean? Put simply it means that there is a 95% chance that a difference found was *real* and not just by chance (or a 5% probability that the findings were accidental and not real). This seems great and almost certain. Think again though. If you have 20 blood tests done and there is a 5% chance that each one will *by chance* be abnormal (or 5% of people who are healthy have the disease), then there is a good chance you would be *abnormal* or someone would be abnormal frequently.

The same thing is true in science. If we do 100 comparisons in a research study (this is common), then we are almost certain to find some *positives*, whether they are real or not. Now, back to our public relations group. They would much rather announce to the world that treatment X was shown to be effective in left-handed men 42 to 45 years old than announce that it was, overall, a complete failure.

To help deal with this, medical journals currently often insist that the analyses that are done be *preplanned* and rational. Why were lefties of a certain age separated? Did the research team plan that in advance, or did they keep chopping up the data until they found somebody that it actually worked for? Unfortunately, violations of this principle occur constantly. The reader can rarely if ever sort this out and the public is almost never given this type of information by the media.

Among the best approaches to these problems is to do what are called *systematic reviews*. These are usually analyses of multiple studies of the same question. The benefit of such reviews is that one can identify findings from multiple small studies that were not apparent from any one study, or decide if a single study showing an effect was an outlier. However, the key is to be sure the correct studies are included in these reviews and that there are no biases, which were included. Notably, some of the largest concerns about the quality and accuracy of systematic reviews are those related to nutrition (Chung et al. 2009).

Therefore, p < 0.05 sounds good, but it proves little by itself in isolation. Furthermore, the opposite is not true either. A p > 0.05 does not mean that it *did not work*. The number of subjects may be too small, there may be isolated *breaches* of the study, and the authors may not have figured out important conflicting factors in the analysis.

There is much more we could say about these issues, but this is not a statistics text. We just want to be sure that no one would expect a single small study to answer big questions or assume that science is easily or fairly represented in the media.

Conducting clinical research that answers meaningful questions about the health of children is a lot of fun to do and very rewarding. We are grateful that we have been able to do such research for many years. But these studies are not inexpensive, fast, or easily replicated. They require expertise not only in the actual study procedures, but also in all aspects of planning and conducting the study.

Even the best plans can fail though. Children may not follow through with what they are supposed to do. Families may move to another city in the midst of a long-term study or families may simply decide to stop participating in a study. This is their absolute right, but when several thousand dollars have been spent on each subject, it is tough when they move out or quit before the end of the study.

It is however, very rewarding when we learn new things from the studies, and we are very grateful to all the children and their families who have participated in our human studies involving bone health. At a minimum, we have studied over a thousand children in the last two decades of human bone health-related research. No complications or injuries have occurred and fewer than a dozen children have withdrawn from the research because they did not tolerate the blood draws or other procedures.

Measuring calcium absorption: How is it really done?

Measuring a child's rate of calcium absorption can be done using many techniques. We'll briefly mention some older methods, and then focus on the current standard, called the *dual-tracer, stable isotope technique*. This is the method we have used for over 20 years involving several thousand subjects, most of them children and adolescents. It is also the method used to measure magnesium and zinc absorption.

Mass balance studies

Historically, calcium absorption was measured using a technique called the *mass balance technique*. In this approach, one measured exactly how much calcium was in the diet for a period of time, usually 7 to 10 days. Then, one collected all of the urine and stool of the research subject for the same length of time. The difference between what went in the body from diet, and what came out in urine and stool, was a measurement of how much was first absorbed, and then retained by the body. Now, this method was, as one can imagine, not very easy to do, especially in small children. For the most part, excluding infants, it has been used in only a few pediatric research studies since the mid-1950s. One group in the United States has continued to use this method with adolescents who stay in a summer camp environment, but few others have done this. This technique requires a prolonged period of time where nearly everything that goes in and comes out of the body is collected, thus usually subjects must be kept in a hospital or outpatient *metabolic ward*. Analyzing the food intake is laborious and collections of urine and stool are often incomplete and unpleasant to collect and chemically analyze.

Some of the results from calcium mass balance studies done prior to World War II are not believable, and although data from studies performed 50 to 80 years ago are widely quoted, these data may not be accurate both due to poor study compliance and inaccurate analytical techniques.

The development of radioactive calcium studies

In the 1950s, a major advance in the ability to measure calcium absorption occurred with the development of radioactive isotope techniques. In this technique, a radioactive calcium tracer was administered by mouth and then after a period of time, the amount of radiation from that dose in the body was measured to determine how much had been absorbed and retained by the body.

An important improvement on this technique came with the development of the dual-tracer method. In this technique, one radioactive tracer of calcium was given by mouth, usually with a small meal, and a different radioactive tracer was given intravenously. The relative recovery of those tracers in urine, or their relative levels in the serum after a period of time, was a very accurate measure of what fraction of the dietary calcium was absorbed. We will not go through the math involved in this, but fundamentally, the dose given intravenously is a correction factor for the dose that is given orally because our bodies do not absorb 100% of the nutrients we eat. After the intravenous tracer is administered, it goes to bone or other tissues before it can be measured. The oral and intravenous tracers go into urine at about the same rate over time. Therefore, the relative amounts of the two tracers in the urine over a time period, usually 24 hours, reflect the dietary absorption of the mineral. No stool or blood samples are needed; just a 24-hour urine collection. In adults, a slight modification of this technique replaces the 24-hour urine collection with a single blood sample drawn several hours after the tracers are given.

This technique does not completely obviate the need for assessment of diet. First, one needs to provide an appropriate diet based on the study design (i.e., high calcium or low phytates) or the subject's usual diet. Second, for many purposes, we are not interested only in the fraction of the dietary calcium that was absorbed which is the value determined directly from the tracer study. We would also like to know the total amount of dietary calcium that is absorbed each day. This amount is the product of the fraction of dietary calcium that is absorbed and the dietary intake of calcium each day. Therefore, accurate assessment of dietary intake is needed while the absorption fraction is being measured.

Performing this dietary assessment can be done in various ways. Most commonly it is done by some method in which a meal is provided on a tray with foods that have been preweighed and whose mineral content is known from food composition tables and software programs. After the meal, any remaining uneaten food is then postweighed and the difference represents the amount of consumed food for each item. Later, the study dietitian determines the nutrient content of the foods consumed and the intake is calculated. There are imperfections in this method, one of which is limitations and inaccuracies in the available food composition tables. Some groups have chemically analyzed food samples as part of their research, but this is uncommon and very expensive.

With some adjustment in sample collection timing, this technique was also applied to other minerals including magnesium and zinc. A huge benefit to this technique is that it does not require long-term food, blood, urine, or stool collections. In fact, most information can be obtained without any stool collection, an obviously appealing aspect to children and adults alike. Not having to collect or measure anything for more than about a day has also made the technique more tolerable than the mass balance technique.

Stable isotope studies of calcium absorption

Although the amounts of radiation subjects receive in radioactive calcium tracer studies is extremely small, it was clearly necessary to find a way to avoid the use of radiation in these tracer studies if this research were to be widely applied to children. To do this, the method of using nonradioactive tracers, called *stable isotopes*, began in the 1960s and was improved and enhanced over the following 20 years. Currently, almost all calcium absorption studies are done using stable rather than radioactive calcium isotopes so as to avoid any radiation exposure to the participating subjects.

A stable isotope is nothing more than a completely naturally occurring form of an element. For this type of research, we are using what are called *minor stable isotopes* of elements such as calcium. What this means is that, in nature, calcium and many other elements have variable amounts of neutrons, and, therefore, variable atomic weights. So, whereas most calcium (over 96%) has 20 neutrons, 20 protons and 20 electrons, and, therefore, has an atomic weight of 40, not all calcium is the same. In fact, every natural source of calcium in the known universe, including moon rocks and asteroids, contains small amounts of calcium that have more than 20 neutrons and exists completely together with the calcium that has 20 neutrons. These are the minor stable isotopes that we administer in our research studies. For example, about 0.6% of all calcium contains 22 neutrons and has an atomic weight of 42. About 2.1% of all calcium has 24 neutrons and an atomic weight of 44.

These minor stable isotopes of calcium exist naturally in all forms of calcium and are biologically identical to the more common calcium with an atomic weight of 40. They have absolutely no radiation release (they are, after all, *stable*) and are completely safe. Clearly, this is safe as they are part of everything that has calcium, from milk to rocks. The use of the term stable isotopes helps families to distinguish them from radioactive isotopes that do release radiation. Henceforth, we will write their names the way scientists do, as ^{40}Ca for calcium with 20 neutrons and an atomic weight of 40, or for the minor isotopes, ^{42}Ca and ^{44}Ca for isotopes with an atomic weight of 42 or 44. There are more minor isotopes of calcium, but ^{42}Ca and ^{44}Ca are often used in human investigations.

Now here is the trick. If we can obtain *pure* or nearly pure ^{42}Ca or ^{44}Ca, we could give it to people, then collect their blood or urine and see if they had increased amounts of ^{42}Ca or ^{44}Ca in these biological samples. If given in the diet, the only way it could get to the blood or urine would be for it to be absorbed, just as with the radioactive isotopes. Furthermore, if we could get two different pure sources of different atomic weight isotopes, such as ^{42}Ca and ^{44}Ca and give one by mouth and one by vein, we could duplicate the radioactive isotope experiments with the huge benefit of not exposing anyone to radiation. A more detailed explanation of this method is provided in these review articles (Abrams 1999; Abrams 2008).

The two great challenges of this are first to obtain the pure or nearly pure ^{42}Ca or ^{44}Ca, and second to actually measure how much of these isotopes, once given, find their way to be absorbed and then excreted in the urine or carried in the blood. Each of these challenges has been a tremendous issue for scientists over the past 40 years. In the case of obtaining the stable isotopes for human research, this must be done after they are purified using a special machine, which is really a gigantic mass spectrometer, called a *calutron*. For any readers who are history buffs, especially those interested in World War II, research this article (Yergey and Yergey 1997) and read about how the calutrons were originally invented for use in purifying uranium for the Manhattan Project during World War II and then came to be used for peaceful purposes, including our stable isotope studies. Here is an excerpt from the article about the use of silver for this wartime effort:

> A Treasury official was approached about the possibility of loaning silver to a wartime emergency project. When the official asked about the amount of silver required, he was told that the project would require about 15,000 tons of the metal. His response was "Sir, we measure our silver in ounces, not tons" [Love 1973]. Despite the official's chagrin, about 300-million Troy ounces of silver were loaned to the Manhattan Engineering District and shipped, under guard, to Detroit for drawing into silver buss. Guards were always present to pick up filings and scrap. After the war, the silver was returned to the Treasury with virtually no loss.

Unfortunately, the only calutrons in the United States, those built for the Manhattan Project, are no longer active. Calcium stable isotopes for our research purposes are currently only made in a few facilities in the former Soviet Union. The isotopes are not cheap, but not beyond what can be purchased for research or even clinical use to measure calcium absorption. To buy enough calcium stable isotopes for a single measurement of calcium absorption costs about $100 to $300 depending on the size and age of the subject. Currently they are purchased via reputable distributers who provide extensive testing of them before sales (http://www.tracesciences.com/ca.htm). All of the stable isotopes must be prepared using appropriate pharmaceutical procedures for dosing either by mouth or by vein and thoroughly tested for safety before being administered.

The good news is that these studies are safe for absolutely anyone. The smallest child we have studied weighed less than two pounds, and we have studied adults up to about 90 years of age with this technique. It is also safe for pregnant and breast-feeding women. The intravenous isotope must be administered in a medically safe way, but the dose of calcium given is extremely tiny and completely safe. There is no meaningful risk to the skin or any other organs from the tiny doses of calcium given when this is done properly using standard sterile techniques. No one has ever been known to be harmed by a calcium stable isotope study since they were first performed over 40 years ago.

Global research of calcium metabolism using stable isotopes

The clinical technique for doing one of these studies is transportable throughout the world. The countries among which we have conducted calcium or zinc stable isotope studies in include Nigeria, Mexico, Peru, Pakistan, India, and Indonesia. Others people have conducted such studies in many more countries around the world. Along with a group of colleagues in Canada, we will be measuring calcium absorption in 2012 in pregnant women in Bangladesh who will be given a calcium supplement.

Although the clinical techniques for this research are transferable almost anywhere, the analytical techniques are not. To take a sample of blood or urine and measure how much of a stable isotope is in it requires special equipment called *mass spectrometers*. Even within the field of mass spectrometry, it requires uncommonly used types of mass spectrometers to measure minerals such as calcium. Therefore, there are relatively few laboratories in the world that perform these analysis and they can be costly. Studies done in most countries have the samples shipped to places where the samples can be analyzed.

A historical note regarding calcium stable isotope studies

The most famous example of a calcium stable isotope study was the one performed on the Space Station Mir. A handful of astronauts and cosmonauts conducted detailed calcium stable isotope studies first while on the ground and later when in space. As you can imagine, it was an incredible logistical challenge to safely administer the isotopes intravenously in space and collect the blood and urine samples (Smith et al. 2005).

Bone loss is an important concern with long-term space flight. Therefore, a further calcium stable isotope study was conducted with the astronauts of *Columbia* STS-107. All samples collected in space from this study were lost with the tragic loss of the shuttle on reentry on February 1, 2003. This PDF file (spaceresearch.nasa.gov/sts-107/107_cal-kin.pdf) contains the preflight description of the STS-107 calcium-related experiment. Another link of interest about the scientists and the project is http://spaceflight.nasa.gov/shuttle/support/people/ssmith.html

Since STS-107, there have been no further calcium stable isotope studies in space and none are currently planned. Some ground-based studies, called bed rest studies, have been done, but it will undoubtedly be a while before calcium or other mineral stable isotopes return to space.

How can a registered dietitian evaluate calcium intake for research studies?

Learning exactly what a person eats and drinks is a challenging task. Various methods of dietary assessments have been validated and are available for registered dietitians (RDs) to use (Burrows, Martin, and Collins 2010). Dietary assessments for research studies depend on the study design, age of the child, and resources available. A nutrition screening is often important for research studies to determine eligibility. Does the potential subject take dietary supplements that are incompatible with the study design? Does the potential subject have any food allergies or intolerances that make her ineligible? A nutrition screening should also evaluate if the potential subject has any special dietary practices that need to be addressed, such as vegetarianism, or if they have what is considered a usual amount of calcium in their dietary choices.

There are several types of dietary assessment, each with its own pros and cons.

1. Basic Dietary History. In this approach, a registered dietitian will ask the subject to describe what they usually eat on a daily basis. *Pros*: Even though it is a basic nutrition history, it can be very comprehensive depending on the time spent. It can include data on the subject's living situation, use of financial assistance programs for food, and supplements consumed. *Cons*: Time-consuming and may or may not be accurate depending on the subject's recall and knowledge of serving sizes.

2. A 24-Hour Dietary Recall. A registered dietitian will ask the subject to describe everything they consumed in the past 24 hours. *Pros*: Most people can remember, especially with some helpful direction, what they ate that recently. It takes very little training for someone to know what to ask, the right questions, and to prompt the most accurate information. *Cons*: The past 24 hours may not have been typical for that person. Was there a celebration? Was it a weekend? Were they feeling ill? Also, sometimes it is hard for a person to accurately describe the portion sizes they ate. Two 24-hour dietary recalls are more accurate than one and provide more information for a general estimate of usual dietary intake. Asking a subject to remember more than 2 days in the past is not accurate or helpful.

3. Food Frequency Questionnaire (FFQ). With this tool, a subject can fill out a worksheet that asks him how often he has eaten particular foods within a set time frame (often a week or month). *Pros*: No training required. For targeting specific nutrients, there are some FFQs that can be found online or otherwise obtained from groups who will share the ones they have used. *Cons*: Some FFQs are quite long

and can take an adult over an hour to complete. Obviously, it is not possible that most children can do this on their own. Some FFQs are nutrient or food specific, and target specifically calcium-rich foods. This provides a good estimate but can leave out lower calcium–containing foods that may be consumed more frequently. In general, we prefer the use of other tools over the use of FFQs, but many large dietary surveys that involve thousands of individuals make use of FFQs.

4. Food Diary. Subjects are asked to write down all the foods and drinks they consume prospectively, often for a 3 to 7 day period. *Pros*: Subjects do not have to rely on their memory to describe what they eat, as with the 24-hour dietary recall. Also, brand names are easily apparent for the subject to write down. *Cons*: A trained professional, usually a dietitian, needs to evaluate the findings and enter them into a nutrient database program to determine the composition of the subject's intake. Subjects need some education on how to measure or estimate food portions, and this can be confusing to many subjects.

5. Weighed Food Diary. The weighed food diary takes a basic food diary to the next level. Subjects are provided with a food scale and trained to weigh their entire dietary intake for a 3-day period. For calcium studies, it is important to know exactly how much of each nutrient is in a food. It is not enough to know just that the subject ate a ham and cheese sandwich, or even that the entire sandwich weighed 250 grams. How much of the 250 grams was the cheese which would be very high in calcium, as opposed to the ham which has very little calcium? As we described in previous chapters, calcium content can vary widely across brands, especially bread. Subjects are instructed to record brand names and weigh food items individually prior to consumption. *Pros*: Very accurate. *Cons*: Time-consuming with expensive labor costs. This method is optimally used in smaller studies such as the stable isotope studies we perform where the best possible estimate of each individual participant's calcium intake is crucial to the success of the study.

After the subject's food and beverage intake has been recorded in some manner, the nutrient composition can be determined. The U.S. Department of Agriculture (USDA) Nutrient Database for Standard Reference (www.nal.usda.gov/fnic/foodcomp/search/) is the basis for virtually all food composition software programs, and includes almost 8000 foods. Some computer programs are free online and offer a limited number of foods and beverages. Other programs are more expensive but offer many more foods as well as nutrients evaluated. The University of Minnesota Nutrition Data System for Research (http://www.ncc.umn.edu/products/ndsr.html) is designed for research studies and is the most accurate software program available, although it is also the most expensive. It includes not only whole foods and combination foods, but also the nutrient composition of store-brand products and fast-food items.

Determining calcium intake during stable isotope studies is best done with a variety of methods. Twenty-four hour dietary recalls are used for screening data to determine if a subject consumes a typical dietary intake of calcium so that the subjects are similar in baseline intake. Cutoffs of 600 mg to 1200 mg calcium per day are often used in our studies to identify small children with unusually low or high intakes. Two days of dietary recalls are mandatory, with a third day being optional if there are any issues with one of the first two days. During the study day in which the subject is receiving stable isotopes or collecting urine for analysis, weighed diet records are best. Using more than one method provides information that may be overlooked if only one method was used, but it does not put too much strain on the subject so that they drop out or become noncompliant.

Summary ideas related to research studies in this area

We hope that this extended discussion of research-related concepts involving bone health will serve two purposes. First, our goal was to inform readers about the challenges of conducting such studies and to help explain why this type of research is not simple, rapid, or inexpensive. Second, we hope to enthuse those who read this to consider involving clinical research in their career. As we noted, the best experimental *model* for the human child is…the human child. Nothing beats conducting safe but meaningful research in the population that you care about!

Becoming a Nutritionally Aware Physician

First of all, this is a great time to plan a career devoted to pediatric nutrition both from a research and a clinical care perspective. People are genuinely interested in providing good nutrition to their children and public awareness of pediatric nutrition, as well as concern about it, is at an all-time high. We have already discussed becoming a dietitian and now we will discuss becoming a physician with an interest in pediatric nutrition. This is not to say that these are the only possibilities. There are plenty of nurses, especially advanced practice nurses, who are very involved in this area as well as physician assistants, and others.

Physicians who are interested in pediatric nutrition are almost always pediatricians. However, pediatric surgeons (an incredible but very long training!) may be closely involved as well. Pediatric surgeons are first trained as surgeons and then specialize in pediatric surgery. They usually do research in their training, and it is not uncommon for it to be a total of 9 years between when they *finish* medical school and when they are practicing independently. This is a long time for any training. Child psychiatrists, who generally first train as psychiatrists and then specialize in pediatrics, are involved in managing children with eating disorders and sometimes this includes being very involved in the nutritional aspects of the management plan.

Among pediatricians, about half will do general community pediatrics and about half will specialize or work in a hospital setting. Training in pediatrics is three years after medical school. Specialty training is an additional three years in most fields.

The two specialty fields most closely connected with pediatric nutrition are pediatric gastroenterology, hepatology, and nutrition; and neonatology (Dr. Abrams' field). In addition, pediatric endocrinologists deal with diabetes, both type 1, juvenile diabetes, and type 2, historically called *adult-onset diabetes*, but it is a form that can occur at any age. Obesity in both children and adults is commonly associated with type 2 diabetes. It is also increasingly a problem managed by pediatric endocrinologists. Pediatric endocrinologists are often called upon to deal with problems such as rickets or other forms of severe bone health problems in children.

In general, neonatologists focus on the care of high-risk infants, especially premature infants. Some will do followup of these infants, which is often heavily nutritionally focused, but currently, most do not do much of the followup. Neonatologists interested in nutrition tend to do research involving human milk, growth of infants, and maternal:infant nutrient interactions. Relatively few neonatologists are experts in nutrition, but those interested in nutrition can certainly make this a focus of their interests.

Pediatric gastroenterologists more generally care for nutritional problems in children of all ages. They deal with many children with chronic illnesses that have nutritional complications, including bone health problems. In particular they are experts in inflammatory bowel disease, allergic bowel disorders, and failure to thrive, a situation in which a child is not growing as expected. They conduct research across the spectrum from basic science studies on the intestine to clinical trials related to nutritional supplementation.

As far as general pediatricians are concerned, there are some who have either special training or expertise in nutrition, but most do not. Pediatric medicine training includes nutrition science, but it is often overwhelmed by the need to learn about infections and other pediatric health problems. As such, there is a huge variation in the knowledge and expertise a pediatrician might have about common nutritional problems such as when to start solid foods and more complex problems such as the nutritional needs of children with cerebral palsy that might be uncommon in their personal practice.

If a physician is really interested in focusing their career on pediatric nutrition, most, but not all, will end up in either neonatology or pediatric gastroenterology, hepatology, and nutrition, although a few may become other types of specialists. There is a large need for more pediatric nutrition experts. In general, very few pediatric physicians in the United States will only do nutrition as their patient care area. In adult medicine and in other countries this can be more common, but it is very uncommon in the United States.

References

Abrams SA. 1999. Using stable isotopes to assess mineral absorption and utilization by children. *Am J Clin Nutr* 70:955–64. A bit of history and a bit of description of how we measure mineral absorption via stable isotopes. This article provides a basic introduction to the technique and its most common applications. (Free online.)

Abrams SA. 2008. Assessing mineral metabolism in children using stable isotopes. *Pediatr Blood Cancer* 50 (2 suppl):438–41. This is a more recent review of the methods for performing mineral stable isotope studies in children. (Not free online.)

Burrows TL, Martin RJ, and Collins CE. 2010. A systematic review of the validity of dietary assessment methods in children when compared with the method of doubly labeled water. *J Am Diet Assoc* 110(10):1501–10. This study evaluated various methods of dietary assessment performed in 15 different studies in over 600 children and compared results to the gold standard of doubly labeled water. Authors discuss the advantages and disadvantages to each method and which one appeared to be the most accurate for children of various ages. All methods have their own drawbacks with over or underestimating food intake. (Free online.)

Chung M, Balk EM, Ip S, Raman G, Yu WW, Trikalinos TA, Lichtenstein AH, Yetley EA, and Lau J. 2009. Reporting of systematic reviews of micronutrients and health: A critical appraisal. *Am J Clin Nutr* 89:1099–113. Nutrition research is amongst the most likely to not be accurately reported, especially when systematic reviews are considered. In other words, do not believe everything you read, even if the author tells you it was *systematically reviewed*. (Free online.)

Lippman SM, Klein EA, Goodman PJ, Lucia MS, Thompson IM, Ford LG, Parnes HL, Minasian LM, Gaziano JM, Hartline JA, Parsons JK, Bearden JD, Crawford ED, Goodman GE, Claudio J, Winquist E, Cook ED, Karp DD, Walther P, Lieber MM, Kristal AR, Darke AK, Arnold KB, Ganz PA, Santella RM, Albanes D, Taylor PR, Probstfield JL, Jagpal TJ, Crowley JJ, Meyskens FL, Baker LH, and Coltman CA Jr. 2009. Effect of selenium and vitamin E on risk of prostate cancer and other cancers: The Selenium and vitamin E Cancer Prevention Trial (SELECT). *JAMA* 301:39–51. A huge study found no effect of selenium with or without vitamin E on prevention of prostate cancer. Afterwards there were plenty who criticized the study design. This always happens with a negative study. (Free online.)

Smith SM, Wastney ME, O'Brien KO, Morukov BV, Larina IM, Abrams SA, Davis-Street JE, Oganov V, and Shackelford LC. 2005. Bone markers, calcium metabolism, and calcium kinetics during extended-duration space flight on the Mir space station. *J Bone Miner Res* 20:208–218. One of the most remarkable human metabolic studies ever conducted happened on the space station Mir. (Not free online.)

Yergey Al and Yergey AK. 1997. Preparative scale mass spectrometry: A brief history of the calutron. *J Am Soc Mass Spec* 8:943–53. An absolutely incredible historical paper related to the calutrons, their role in the Manhattan project, and their later conversion to peaceful uses such as mineral stable isotope studies. The article, written by Dr. Abrams' mentor (and recently his daughter, Hannah's, mentor), Alfred Yergey, Ph.D., and his son, Karl, includes some remarkable historical pictures of a time and place that changed our history. (Free online.)

chapter fourteen

Programming and genetics

Does milk make a child grow tall?

One reason often quoted for making sure that children of all ages get enough calcium and vitamin D, especially in the form of milk, is to make sure they grow tall. We intuitively believe that our children will be taller if they drink lots of milk that contains the calcium needed for growth. Few take note that there are plenty of children who never drink milk who have quite normal growth patterns. We are not vegans nor are we opponents of milk, but we also do not agree with any attempt to scare people into drinking cow's milk who truly wish to avoid it for themselves or their children.

The reality, therefore, is that the belief that milk will make a child grow tall is *sort of* true. In the late 19th and early 20th century, it was demonstrated that adding milk to the diet of undernourished children improved their height growth. More recently, there are cases in which undernourished children have a marked improvement in growth when provided a healthy diet including dairy products.

However, it is probably not really the calcium and vitamin D that are making most of the difference for the majority of these children. Poor height growth is primarily related to protein and energy deficiency, not bone mineral deficiency, although this can play a role. We each have a genetically determined height, and it may even be that we absorb calcium in order to get enough bone minerals to support the bones we grow (Abrams JCEM 2005). If we are energy deficient, and especially protein deficient, we might not reach that programmed height.

For most children, as long as they have enough protein and energy in their diet, increasing their calcium intake itself, through dairy or other means, will not make them taller than they are programmed to become by their genetics. Phrased another way, parents who are each 5 feet 6 inches should not expect their sons or daughters to be 6 feet tall if they drink a lot of milk or take calcium supplements. Studies clearly indicate that most of one's final height is related to genetic programming, not our diet.

An interesting exception to this is children with very severe growth failure associated with rickets. In this condition, although the bones are growing, they are not mineralized adequately. Therefore, the bones become bowed and height is inadequate. This improves with treatment, but some genetically programmed height might be lost. Rickets is not a benign condition, and we need to emphasize the importance of adequate vitamin D intake and calcium in its prevention.

One of the most important new areas of investigation related to nutrition is the role our genetic makeup plays in determining our body composition and the values of nutrients in our blood and tissues. For example, as we have noted African-Americans have a greater bone mineral density despite lower calcium intakes and lower vitamin D levels than Caucasians. This difference is clearly apparent in childhood after the first few years of life and persists through adulthood. Genetically mediated differences in handling of calcium in the intestines and kidneys may be the major aspect of this difference. Males have less osteoporosis than females although about 20% of osteoporosis cases occur in males.

More recently, scientists have been interested in determining exactly what genes control things like bone mineralization, height, and even calcium absorption. The idea is that if we can identify specific genes regulating the process of bone growth or bone loss, then we can both identify at-risk individuals for more close screening, and develop and test specific interventions.

Of course, this is much easier said than done, and although relatively free of ethical concerns, still needs to be understood in terms of the relative benefits of the information to the individual versus the risks of having such information be known. We are always concerned about labeling individuals as being likely to develop a health disorder that will be costly and how that might affect their health insurance or job opportunities.

First, however, let's consider the science involved. Beginning about 20 years ago, scientists began to identify genes that were related to bone health. Since then, many such genes have been identified and numerous large studies performed to evaluate the relationship between different genes, the forms of the genes people have and outcomes related to bone.

Overall, just like for many diseases (cancer) or even nutritional issues (obesity), the results have been a bit confusing and inconsistent. There is little doubt that some specific genes are associated with bone mineralization and loss. These genes are primarily those related to what is called the *Vitamin D Receptor protein* (VDR). The VDR protein is an intracellular protein that when bound to the active form of vitamin D forms a transcription factor that ultimately affects many cellular processes (Fleet and Schoch 2010). In other words, this protein allows vitamin D to make lots of important things happen in the body. Although the best known of these effects are those leading to increased calcium absorption, it is also involved in the absorption of phosphorus as well as many other effects.

We have found that one gene related to the vitamin D receptor expression, called the *fok1 gene*, has forms called *polymorphisms* that are directly related to calcium absorption in young adolescents. This same gene has been associated with a variety of biological effects, including some related to cancer. Adolescents with one form of the gene have much higher rates of calcium absorption than those with a different form (Abrams JBMR 2005). Animal research supports this relationship (Xue and Fleet 2009).

As of now, we really do not have a good idea how to use this type of information in a clinical setting. We just do not have enough information to tailor dietary requirements to specific genes. On the whole, this is currently just information of value for researchers. This will undoubtedly change in the future when we identify a large enough pattern of genes affecting a range of nutritional outcomes and learn how our diet interacts with them. Whether we will be able to identify genetic patterns of bone formation and risk of osteoporosis leading to specific effective interventions is far from certain.

Ultimately, the field of gene-nutrient interactions, in which we look at an individual's genetics and then try to determine the best nutrient intake for each individual based on their genetic makeup will be important. At present, however, despite the enthusiasm of some for using genetic information to set nutritional guidelines, we are not really quite at that point yet. Perhaps, we will be in the next 5 to 10 years, however.

Keep an eye out also for the field of epigenetics. This is an area of research in which nonchromosomal effects on genetic material may be involved in determining nutritional and other important biological outcomes. For example, Suter et al. (2011) recently reported using a primate model where exposure to a maternal high-fat diet *in utero* significantly altered the expression of fetal hepatic gene expression. In other words, what you eat during pregnancy can effect how genes work in your body. This field of work is in its earliest form, but represents part of the new world of relating genetics to diet and nutritional status.

References

Abrams SA, Griffin IJ, Hawthorne KM, and Liang L. 2005; Height and height Z-score are related to calcium absorption in 5- to 15 year-old girls. *J Clin Endocrinol Metab* 90:5077–81. How tall a child grows can be related to how much calcium they absorb. The question is, "which drives which?" We think it is most likely that you are genetically programmed to a height and then absorb the calcium you need to reach that height unless your calcium intake is markedly deficient. Interestingly, these same relationships exist in studies in adults as well. (Free online.)

Abrams SA, Griffin IJ, Hawthorne KM, Chen Z, Gunn SK, Wilde W, Darlington G, Shypailo R, and Ellis K. 2005 Vitamin D receptor Fok1 polymorphisms affect calcium absorption, kinetics and bone mineralization rates during puberty. *J Bone Miner Res* 20:945–53. We found that genetic differences related to one gene involved in vitamin D regulation affected both the ability of the body to absorb calcium and also the bone mineralization of the bones in pubertal children. (Not free online.)

Fleet JC and Schoch RD. 2010 Molecular mechanisms for regulation of intestinal calcium absorption by vitamin D and other factors. *Crit Rev Clin Lab Sci* 47:181–95. A detailed review of the relationship between calcium absorption and genetic and hormonal factors, including the vitamin D receptor. (Not free online.)

Suter M, Bocock P, Showalter L, Hu M, Shope C, McKnight R, Grove K, Lane R, and Aagaard-Tillery K. 2011 Epigenomics: Maternal high-fat diet exposure *in utero* disrupts peripheral circadian gene expression in nonhuman primates. *FASEB J* 25:714–26. The cutting edge of the relationship between genetics, epigenetic phenomenon, and nutrition as reflected in this study of pregnancy in nonhuman primates. (Not free online.)

Xue Y, and Fleet JC. 2009. Intestinal vitamin D receptor is required for normal calcium and bone metabolism in mice. *Gastroenterology* 136:1317–27. Although this is in an animal model, the ideas are clear and the data helpful in understanding the human relationship between vitamin D receptors and bone mineral metabolism. (Free online.)

chapter fifteen

Frequently asked questions

1. Does it matter when a child is given his calcium supplement?

First, remember that it is generally best to provide calcium to children as part of their regular diet, not as a supplement. Children need lots of nutrients for growth and calcium is only one of them. Therefore, consider that dairy products and many vegetables are great natural sources of calcium, and other foods and beverages, such as cereals and orange juice are fortified with calcium.

Most children who receive a calcium supplement will either get a relatively small supplement pill, usually no more than 500 mg per day, or will receive their daily supplemental calcium, not uncommonly about 200 to 250 mg, as part of a once daily multivitamin, multimineral supplement. It is best to give supplements with a meal, and it is often easiest to remember to give vitamins and supplements with breakfast. However, the effect of timing is generally not that crucial for most children. Supplements containing 200 to 250 mg calcium taken once or twice daily are not big enough to substantially decrease calcium absorption by overwhelming the calcium absorptive mechanisms of the body. They will not have a substantial long-term effect on the absorption of other key nutrients either.

The bottom line is to find the time that works best for each child. Taking a supplement with a meal is ideal, but it is not so crucial as to make much difference. Some children and adolescents remember best to do things when they wake up with breakfast, others remember better in the evening with or after dinner. Some never remember to take out the trash, empty the dishwasher, or take a vitamin and mineral supplement.

2. Does it matter when I give my child his vitamin D?

There are remarkably few studies that evaluate, in any age group, the best timing for giving vitamin D supplements. For infants who are breast-fed, if they are receiving any bottles of mother's milk, such as when the mother is at work, then the vitamin–containing drops can be mixed in with the breast milk. If the mother is pumping her breast milk, during the first weeks of life it is best to go with only breast-feeding, and save the bottle of mother's milk until the breast-feeding is well established. For babies who are only feeding at the breast, it can be a bit challenging to get the baby to take the dropper of vitamins, but they can be squeezed right into the infant's mouth.

There are some vitamin D drops that are designed and marketed for placement directly on the breast, and then ingested by the infant while nursing. This is an interesting idea, but we would like to see published data about how readily this works for most babies in terms of the quantity of absorbed vitamin D. Still, for those babies who spit out any other way of giving the drops, this is a consideration that might be worth a try.

For older children receiving cow's milk or other milk type beverages, it is reasonable to mix a liquid vitamin supplement in with the milk to disguise it a bit. For children old enough to take a gummy, chewable tablet, or pill, it does not matter that much. Vitamin D is usually absorbed with fat, so taking it with a regular meal is reasonable, but for healthy children it probably does not make much difference. Children who do not absorb nutrients very well, such as those with cystic fibrosis or Crohn's disease, might benefit from taking vitamin D supplements with meals for better absorption. They should also consider taking water-soluble versions of vitamin D. These are vitamins that are specially formulated so that they do not need fat to be absorbed. It is best to discuss these situations with a dietitian, pharmacist, or physician who is specifically experienced with vitamin supplementation in children with the specific health concern involved.

3. Is it okay to give calcium with iron?

This is an interesting question and one about which we have done several research studies. Also, it is a good example of where science can be misleading in relation to nutrition.

It has been known and shown for many decades that there is competition between some minerals in the gut, such that if an individual takes calcium with iron, the calcium gets absorbed and much of the iron does not. In a similar way, there is competition for absorption between iron and zinc. Sometimes, this works in a positive way. Some data suggest that high intakes of calcium compete with toxic minerals such as lead for absorption, and that high calcium intakes can decrease lead toxicity. Other clinical data are somewhat more equivocal about this effect in a practical sense as an approach to decreasing lead toxicity.

However, what is true in an isolated scientific experiment is not always true when applied to a real long-term diet. What several research groups, including ours, have reported is that if someone takes supplemental calcium with iron over a long period of time, say six weeks or more, this effect completely disappears. That is, there is no harm to the iron absorption from taking it with calcium.

So, all of that wise advice not to take iron with milk, or to separate pills with calcium from those with iron is not really necessary. For the most part, people can have their milk with their iron-fortified breakfast cereal and not be concerned about it. They can even have a nice Texas steak with a glass of milk, as long as they are not trying to keep kosher and separating meat and milk, in which case it should be a nice lean brisket with some calcium-fortified orange juice to drink!

4. Does it matter what form of calcium supplement a child receives?

For most children it does not make much difference. Calcium citrate has some potential benefits for those who have less gastric acid, including some elderly individuals and some children with chronic illnesses. However, for most children after 4 to 6 months of age, the less expensive calcium carbonate will be absorbed well. It can be difficult clinically to determine whether an individual will malabsorb calcium given as calcium carbonate so discussion with an expert related to a child's specific condition is warranted. Infants rarely require home calcium supplementation, but when they do, it is generally best not to use calcium carbonate due to their relatively high stomach pH.

Calcium absorption fraction, that is, the efficiency with which most children absorb calcium after infancy, is about 30% of the intake. During puberty, it increases to 40% to 45%, after which it drops back to about 30% postpuberty. It stays at about that rate until about age 50 years or so when it gradually drops to 20% to 25%. During pregnancy, calcium absorption goes up to 50% to 60% in most women, sometimes slightly higher.

5. Chocolate milk: Friend or foe?

This is one of the most controversial issues related to bone mineral rich foods for children. There is a major battle between those who would like to have chocolate milk included in school lunches and those who want it banned. In considering this, we first want to remind you that one of us (SAA) serves as a scientific advisor for the Milk Processors Education Program (MilkPep). MilkPep not unexpectedly is strongly in favor of allowing chocolate milk in schools and in the diet as a key source of calcium and vitamin D.

Understanding this issue requires consideration of what, if any, harm might exist in allowing children to have chocolate milk at home when not yet in school, and in preschools and beyond. This consideration must

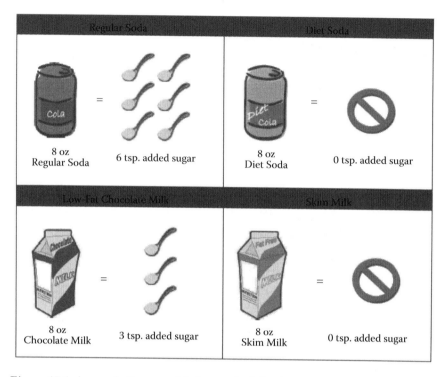

Figure 15.1 Amount of sugar added to typical drinks consumed by children.

include evaluating what would happen to the diets of these children if chocolate milk were to be excluded both at home and in schools, especially if removed from publicly provided school lunches. The potential harm in providing chocolate milk is that it has more calories and more sugar than white (unflavored) milk. There is no added sugar in unflavored milk, but low-fat chocolate milk has up to 3 teaspoons of added sugar (per 8 ounces). It definitely does add calories, but fewer calories than in a regular soft drink (Figure 15.1). Currently the milk producers of the United States are actively working on developing good tasting lower calorie and lower sugar–containing chocolate milks as well as low-fat or fat-free chocolate milk, on average, flavored milk has 30% less added sugar now compared to just 5 years ago. The ones we have sampled are tasty; but, they might take a bit of time to get used to just like any similar change in our diet.

The second concern is that getting small children used to having chocolate milk as their milk is more likely to make them not drink white milk, and, therefore, to have a long-term diet with flavored and thus higher sugar–containing milk. Certainly, we have learned to become used to less salt in our diet so it is reasonable that we can get used to drinking white milk instead of chocolate milk.

The reality is obvious to parents, school dietitians, teachers, and any-one else that cares to talk to children that they overwhelmingly prefer to have the option of chocolate milk be available at home and especially at school. Take chocolate milk away from schools and milk consumption drops 35% on average, a decline that still is not recovered 1 to 2 years later. We will almost certainly find increased consumption of energy drinks and sodas with overall lower intakes of calcium and vitamin D. One can try to ban energy drinks and sodas from school machines, but this is a challenging task that should be considered separately from the chocolate milk issue. The decrease in overall milk consumption when chocolate milk is removed as an option has been shown in well-per-formed research studies, and although such findings are controversial, this is almost certainly a real phenomenon.

School contract negotiators have been under immense pressure in the past decade to follow new guidelines related to the availability of sodas to children during the school day. Often vending machines can only oper-ate before or after school and definitely not during lunch. Although these efforts have been somewhat successful, this too is not the sole answer for increasing calcium and vitamin D intakes in children. Banning all fla-vored milks from schools will unquestionably have an effect on the intake of these key nutrients.

Many school districts encourage milk drinking by having a *flavor of the week*. This gives the children variety so that they learn to develop wider taste preferences as well as it excites children about a healthy bever-age. You would be surprised what kind of flavors children like best—not just chocolate, but also blueberry, pina colada, and triple berry!

So, what do we recommend? Well, this is one of those unsolv-able conundrums in which we have to balance legitimate compet-ing concerns. We do not support banning flavored milk from schools or at home. But, we do think that it should be low-fat chocolate milk (preferably 1% or less) as well as the lower sugar–containing choco-late milk options as these become more available in the marketplace. Furthermore, it is important for parents to try to get their children to choose both low-fat white milk (1% or less for most children over age 2) and low-fat chocolate milk. As children head through the elementary school years, it is important to emphasize white milk with breakfast and meals. But, we should not force away all of the chocolate milk, especially the low-fat versions from our schools, in what will not be a successful attempt to prevent or treat childhood obesity at the expense of other important health needs.

We would rather see children drinking low fat or fat-free flavored milk than throwing white milk into the trash. Food is not nutritional if it is thrown away.

6. Can I choose any brand of calcium supplement?

Certainly, one should only choose sources that are trustworthy *not* to be contaminated with toxic substances including lead and mercury. So, be cautious. Supplements should come from a reputable manufacturer with a record of safe production verified by independent groups. See Chapter 5 for more discussion regarding multivitamins.

Supplement sources that are mostly candy or chocolate are hard to categorize. An occasional treat is fine for any child. However, there is no reason to teach children that candy is the way to receive healthy nutrients. We have nothing against child-friendly products like gummies, but we do not recommend relying on high sugar–containing cereals or candy bars to deliver key nutrients.

7. Should supplements be used that contain magnesium as well as calcium?

We have not mentioned magnesium much in this book. Magnesium is an important factor in bone health. For the most part, diets of small children have plenty of well-absorbed magnesium. It is more common for adolescents than small children to have a diet with not enough magnesium. There is extremely little research that has been done into the magnesium requirements of small children. Magnesium may have many health benefits beyond bone health including reducing headaches and high blood pressure. Please support more magnesium research because we like doing it and think it is important and undervalued.

Therefore, as with other nutrients, the best thing to do is identify natural magnesium sources first. The best sources of magnesium are legumes (black-eyed peas), nuts (and nut butters), whole grains, and some green vegetables. Foods are rarely fortified with magnesium with the exception of breakfast cereals (See Table 4.7).

Be cautious about providing children more than 100 to 200 mg per day of magnesium supplement in pill or liquid supplement form. Most multivitamins do not exceed these amounts, and it would be uncommon to take in large amounts of magnesium from most vitamin supplements.

8. Is it acceptable to allow a small child to drink coffee? What about diet soda?

There are some cultures in which coffee is introduced into the diet of weaning infants. In general, coffee is not a great nutrient source for infants and small children. It displaces other healthy beverages that contain important nutrients. But when discussing coffee, most of the concern is usually about the caffeine and whether caffeine is harmful for bones. Caffeine may cause something called *calciuria,* which just means an increase in calcium in the urine. Caffeine does not really block intestinal absorption of calcium, although that is often claimed. The effect however, on calcium in the urine is real, but usually relatively small. One or two cups of coffee a day will not make your bones go away.

Nonetheless, it is hard to see why chocolate milk is pilloried and coffee is exalted in the diets of teenagers. These days many teenagers live at the local coffee shop consuming coffee day and night. Do we want adolescents to use caffeine to stay up all night to study for the SATs so they can get the 2400 they think they need for Harvard, or the 800 in Math Level 2 they might need for the much better school in Cambridge, Massachusetts (also known as Massachusetts Institute of Technology [MIT], Dr. Abrams' alma mater and his daughter's current university)? Moderate coffee drinking, especially among social teenagers at local coffee shops, will not have a big effect on bones.

With regard to soda, especially diet soda, the pros and cons are even more difficult to evaluate. In general, *dark* sodas contain phosphorus. We have discussed that phosphorus is important for healthy bone formation; but, in excess, along with the acid of sodas, it can cause bone loss. However, the amount of phosphorus in one or two cans of a dark soda is small relative to overall dietary phosphorus and very unlikely to cause much problem. In adults, the data support the idea that small amounts of soda are not problematic for bones. The data in teenagers are not as clear and there are essentially no data in younger children. As noted, the acid load of carbonated beverages may also be a concern. Again, this has not been shown to have much effect at moderate levels and is hardly a major issue overall for teenagers and children.

On the whole, the message of moderation works well here. Children and adolescents do not need coffee or diet soda or energy drinks. Ban these, however, and you might find them drinking things that are worse, or they will just drink them anyway when parents are not looking. Emphasize water and milk and then moderation in all other things.

9. How will oral contraceptives affect the bones of an adolescent?

Many adolescent girls are taking some form of hormonal agents including estrogens. Sometimes this is related to menstrual irregularities and sometimes for contraceptive purposes. The effects of estrogens are generally positive related to bone health and there is little or no need to be concerned about this. In the situation of a girl with menstrual irregularities related to an eating disorder or some athletes, it is worth discussing this with her doctor to see if hormonal use might be indicated along with a comprehensive diet plan. A bone density measurement may be needed along with a complete medical history and physical exam.

10. If a child is from a religious tradition that dresses in clothing that covers most of the arms, legs, or face, does that affect the best choices of minerals and vitamins for them?

There are lots of people who wear clothing that covers most or all of their arms and legs or leaves only small amounts of their face and neck exposed to sunlight. Some of these people are also from ethnic and racial groups with dark skin. This near total skin covering unquestionably has a major effect on vitamin D conversion from solar exposure and this should be considered in nutritional planning. Extremely low serum 25(OH)D levels are routinely reported in women who dress in this fashion and sometimes the levels may be low enough in pregnant women to cause very low serum vitamin D and possibly serum calcium levels in their newborns.

The Institute of Medicine (IOM) dietary guidelines should be followed for all children and adults who have very limited sunshine exposure to their skin due to their clothing. Although routine measurement of serum 25(OH)D levels is not currently advocated in this population, in some cases, especially if there is a clinical reason to suspect bone health problems, such as clinical evidence of early rickets, this might be advisable. Targeting vitamin D intakes slightly higher than 600 IU per day in adolescents might also be reasonable for this group, although there is no evidence that routine doses of several thousand IU each day are needed and considerably more research is needed to determine the best approach to vitamin D intake in this population.

11. What about pregnant women and vitamin D?

This has been covered in Chapter 7 in some detail. In summary, there is no strong evidence for a benefit to additional vitamin D during pregnancy beyond the IOM recommended amounts. It is important to have an appropriate vitamin D intake during pregnancy of about 600 IU per day. Some obstetricians may reasonably recommend an additional supplement of 500 to 1500 IU per day, and this is likely safe, although there is no strong evidence for a specific health outcome benefit for mother or infant.

An area of some interest and inadequate data are the needs of pregnant adolescents. Pregnant adolescents may still be in the latter part of forming their own bones while also providing for their baby. Evidence for a benefit for high-dose minerals or vitamins is lacking, but certainly attention should be paid to this high-risk group.

12. If a baby was born a month early, does he need extra calcium or vitamin D when home from the hospital?

It is often recommended that very premature infants, especially those born at less than 32 weeks gestation or less than about 4 pounds be given extra calcium when they go home. This was discussed in Chapter 3. If formula-fed, this is generally done by providing special high-mineral formulas designed for premature infants for a period of time. For breast-fed infants, sometimes feeding one or two bottles per day of one of these formulas is recommended. In other cases, the breast-fed baby is watched carefully for growth. There is no evidence that preterm babies need more vitamin D than term infants, although because they take in less formula, sometimes vitamin D is given as a supplement even to formula-fed babies to ensure they receive a full 400 IU per day.

For bigger preterm babies, such as those born 3 to 6 weeks early (often called *late preterm infants*), there is less evidence for any special calcium requirements. It is probably the case that no higher intakes of calcium or vitamin D are needed beyond what is recommended for full-term infants. If exclusively fed human milk, then it is important that vitamin D drops be started as early as possible, preferably in the first few days of life.

13. Will participation in high school football affect a child's calcium or vitamin D requirement?

This is certainly an interesting question. There is relatively little information about specific dietary calcium or vitamin D for competitive athletes, including football players. A few have claimed health benefits from high-dose vitamin D supplementation, but this has not been evaluated in any systematic way.

However, it is true that athletes have increased bone mineral content, and, therefore, they need more calcium to build their bones. What we do not really know is whether the Recommended Dietary Allowances (RDAs) for calcium and vitamin D are enough for athletes such as football players, or whether extra would be beneficial. Certainly, many athletes will have fairly high calcium intakes from drinking lots of milk or eating a lot of cheese and pizza products. The new Tolerable Upper Intake Levels (UL) for calcium took this into account.

The bottom line is that it is reasonable to try to ensure that football players at least reach the 1300 mg per day calcium intake and 600 IU per day vitamin D intake. It is possible that a bit more than that would be even better, but there is not any evidence to support megadosing of calcium or vitamin D for any type of athlete.

14. What about gymnasts or runners? Will these sports affect a child's needs for calcium or vitamin D?

In general, there is little likelihood that intakes that substantially exceed the RDAs will be beneficial here either. Furthermore, it is important to recognize that using vitamin and mineral supplements for girls who have exercise-induced menstrual irregularities and/or eating disorders will not solve their bone problems. In the presence of these problems, calcium is not well-absorbed or used properly for bone mineralization. Recognizing that 10% of individuals with disordered eating are males, appropriate physical and mental treatments are necessary.

Excluding this situation, the best suggestion is to ensure an RDA intake of minerals and vitamins, and to focus on diet, not supplements, as much as possible.

15. How can lactose-intolerant children get enough calcium and vitamin D?

This is an extremely common question. Many people have some degree of intolerance to lactose. However, this is a condition that can be over-diagnosed and overtreated as well. Many people who get a mild upset stomach or gas with milk will do fine with other dairy products or with limiting the size of each serving. Those who do have a problem with milk or dairy can often do well with lactose-free milk products or a range of products that can be used to help with lactose intolerance. Milk that has had the lactase enzyme added to it is widely available in grocery stores. In addition, if a lactose-intolerant individual would still like to enjoy dairy products she can take lactase enzymes in pill form with meals to aid in digestion. Nondairy sources of calcium are also important. These include fortified soy and other types of nondairy milk as well as calcium and vitamin D–containing foods such as breakfast cereals.

So, there are plenty of dietary options before resorting to pill or other supplements. Although these may certainly be used, it is worthwhile trying to see if some of the other dietary approaches can be used first. Read Chapters 5 and 6 for some other sources of calcium and vitamin D.

16. How can a mother be sure that her breast milk has enough calcium for her infant?

The good news is that for babies at or near full-term, breast milk undoubtedly has enough calcium for the baby. Rickets does not occur when babies are breast-fed as long as they have enough vitamin D. It is a good idea for lactating women to make sure they are getting adequate calcium at the level of the RDA, but increasing the mother's calcium does not directly translate into more calcium in breast milk. The amount of calcium in breast milk is fairly tightly regulated regardless of a woman's diet.

After six months of age, it is advisable to provide infants with some calcium–containing solid foods to supplement breastfeeding. However, large amounts of calcium are not needed in the supplemental food. A common mixture of foods will usually suffice. A slight delay in introducing solid foods beyond six months will not be harmful to bones as long as vitamin D is provided.

17. Are artificial sweeteners acceptable for children? How much is too much?

This is a very controversial issue in pediatric nutrition right now. For otherwise healthy children, an occasional beverage or other food with artificial sweeteners is almost certainly nonproblematic. It is nearly impossible to stop children from having some diet sodas. Sometimes, it amazes us that some parents will give their teenagers a beer but worry about the health effects of a can of diet soda. There is no connection between artificial sweeteners and bone health within reasonable intakes.

Parents need to sometimes fight with their children about completing their homework on time and staying out late. Allowing them a can of diet soda every once in a while is reasonable, and parents should know that their children's bones can handle it. Note that there is no evidence that drinking diet sodas will do anything to help weight control and some recent evidence suggests, but does not prove, that it may make weight control worse. Regardless, moderation is the key.

18. What can be done to make sure a child with cow's milk protein allergy gets enough calcium and vitamin D?

It is important to distinguish true cow's milk protein allergy or intolerance from lactose intolerance. An allergy to cow's milk protein is a much more serious condition and usually requires careful monitoring by a pediatrician or allergy specialist. In the case of a true protein allergy, dairy is generally not tolerated, and calcium and vitamin D will need to come from other nondairy sources. Sometimes, this gets better with time, but should be managed by an expert such as a pediatric gastroenterologist.

However, some of these nondairy sources include fortified foods and juices, so not all of the calcium and vitamin D needs to come from a supplement. Using nondairy milk will depend on the child, and it needs to be discussed with the pediatrician or allergy specialist.

19. How does being overweight affect a child's serum 25(OH)D levels? Do overweight or obese children need more vitamin D supplementation?

Overweight children generally have lower serum 25(OH)D levels and these levels are probably lowest in the most overweight children. Right now, there is a lot of controversy about how to interpret these levels, and what to do about them. It appears that some of the vitamin D is being stored in the adipose (fat) tissue and that when people lose weight, it gets released from these tissues into the bloodstream where it can be measured.

There is also interest in the idea that low vitamin D levels might make children and adults more likely to develop diabetes. The evidence for this is, as yet, inconclusive. Nonetheless, it is uncertain whether high doses of vitamin D, needed to assure that overweight children get to the same serum level of 25(OH)D in their blood as non-overweight children, are needed. It is also not certain whether frequent blood tests to measure serum 25(OH)D have benefits for these children.

Currently, we recommend that overweight children and adolescents receive at least 600 IU per day of vitamin D and perhaps a bit more up to 1000 to 1200 IU per day although there is no evidence at all that doses above the RDA have specific clinical health benefits for overweight or obese children, and adolescents. Very high doses, especially those over 4,000 IU per day have not been shown to be beneficial and should be limited to special cases determined by a physician with careful monitoring.

20. How does cooking affect vitamins and minerals in the food?

For the most part, cooking does not really affect the bone minerals and vitamin D. Some foods such as fish and eggs have vitamin D, but heat does not destroy the majority of vitamin D in the food. Calcium is also not particularly affected by heating. After all, moderate heat does not really make a mineral go away. So go ahead and enjoy a veggie pizza with melted mozzarella cheese and irradiated mushrooms with extra vitamin

D and know that the nutrients you want are not going to be destroyed in the oven.

21. What is the difference between enriched and fortified?

This is more of a technical distinction that does not make any difference once the food enters your body. *Enriched* means that nutrients that were naturally occurring in the product but were removed during processing (such as with wheat bread) were added back by the manufacturer at the end. *Fortified* means that the manufacturer added nutrients to the food that were never there to begin with such as with calcium-fortified orange juice or vitamin C-fortified apple juice. Neither the calcium in the orange juice, nor the vitamin C in apple juice, was part of the natural product in significant amounts.

22. Why do tortillas have calcium in them?

To get a great calcium containing tortilla you have to go to Mexico. Well, or go to a Tex-Mex restaurant! There, the corn masa (dough) is mixed with water containing lime (lime from limestone, not lime from the fruit), which is actually high in calcium. Since we know that moderate heating does not destroy calcium, the final product retains the calcium added in the processing.

Several national brands of tortillas available in grocery stores have calcium in them, either due to calcium propionate used as a preservative or the use of lime in the processing of the white or yellow corn masa flour, or both. Commercially sold corn tortillas may have 20 to 40 mg calcium each while flour tortillas may have 100 to 200 mg calcium.

23. Many children like frozen yogurt (Fro Yo) more than regular yogurt. How are they different nutritionally and what is the better choice?

Frozen yogurt typically has less calcium than regular yogurt, and usually does not contain vitamin D. It sometimes has slightly more or added sugar. It also lacks the live active cultures that regular yogurt is known for which are helpful for digestive health and bacterial flora. Differences in fiber intake compared with regular yogurt can be decreased if you add some fresh fruit to your frozen yogurt. Evaluating frozen yogurts is another reason why one needs to read food labels since the nutrient content will vary considerably by brand. As yogurt shops become increasingly widespread, we expect makers of frozen yogurts to more often add things like vitamin D and live, active cultures to their products.

24. What are prebiotics? Probiotics? Functional foods?

The term *functional food* is one commonly used to mean a food that is thought to have a positive affect on a specific health benefit based on its often less primary components. Lots of fruits and vegetables (e.g., pomegranates) and juices made from them are in this category. Sometimes, the nutrient may occur naturally in the food, such as the phytonutrient lycopene in tomatoes that has been suggested to decrease the risk of prostate cancer. Other times, the nutrient is added to the product. Calcium and vitamin D-fortified orange juice is an example of this. Each of those products is considered a functional food because it offers an additional health benefit that goes beyond their traditional value.

Notably, some of the benefits ascribed to functional foods are probably real; some are probably not. A lot of research is going into this area right now. Be cautious of what you believe from this literature and be aware that the descriptive phrase, *functional food,* is not regulated by the Food and Drug Administration (FDA). Some of the research on functional foods is funded by various groups with a financial tie to the marketing of these products and may not be unbiased in its interpretation.

Specifically, there is interest in functional foods that affect the bacteria in our intestinal tract. Most people do not like to think about this but we share our bodies with a whole lot of bacteria. Some of them are friendly and some are not so friendly (think acne). However, we can, through what we eat, affect what bacteria are in our intestine, and it may be that we can do so in ways that improve our health.

Probiotics are beneficial bacteria added to foods and are thought to be helpful for us. Probiotics are typically found in yogurt, but also can be found in some milk types including a few commercial infant formulas. In contrast, *prebiotics* are actually carbohydrates that affect the composition of our intestinal flora. This is the *food* that the live bacteria (probiotics) thrive on in order to reproduce and flourish. The most well known prebiotic is a substance called *inulin* found naturally in chicory roots, bananas, and onions. The term *symbiotic* is used when a food contains both probiotics and prebiotics.

Many health benefits have been associated with probiotics and prebiotics. This includes not just intestinal health but possible effects on cardiovascular health. In relation to bone health, we have reported that some prebiotics increase the absorption of calcium from the diet. That is not the most important reason to look for foods with prebiotics, but is a bonus that can be of some value. Wouldn't you like to absorb even more calcium from that cup of yogurt if you could? Is it worth it to pay more for a food with prebiotics just to absorb more calcium? Maybe not, but the whole spectrum of health benefits from prebiotics may make this a reasonable choice.

25. Is it a bad idea to give soymilk to children because of the isoflavone level and possible hormone effects?

No, this is not true. Soymilk is safe and will not cause problems related to hormones in boys or girls. Soymilks, made from soybeans, naturally contain isoflavones that are structurally similar to estrogen. However, there have been no health problems in children because of this. Infants who are exclusively fed soy formula do not have any hormonal changes due to soy intake.

However, soymilks are not always ideal sources of calcium, and not all soymilks are fortified with calcium and vitamin D. In some studies, the calcium is not as well-absorbed from these milks compared to cow's milk. Still even at half or two-thirds the calcium absorption rate, it is better than unfortified soymilk, so it is worthwhile trying to choose fortified soymilks over unfortified ones. Soymilk comes in a variety of flavors and fat levels (whole milk, low-fat, and skim milk). The amount of protein might be slightly lower than a glass of cow's milk but not enough to really worry about.

26. Aren't there hormones in milk that are not healthy for children? Isn't organic milk a better choice?

This is another huge controversy and thousands of articles have been written on this on both sides of the issue. We think that everyone should make his own choice after reviewing the literature. One of us (SAA) does not routinely choose organic milk unless it is his family's favorite brand at the time based on flavor, while one of us (KMH) always purchases it for use at home. That tells you what you need to know about our opinion on this. Families can reasonably make choices for health reasons, taste, frequency, and amount that their family drinks, as well as social reasons related to their view on farming and animal care. Sometimes, too, organic manufacturers are at the leading edge of the best tasting, lower sugar, and lower fat products, or, products with pre and probiotics. Therefore, there are lots of things for consumers to consider in making these decisions.

Milk is a natural substance. Because it comes from a living organism, it contains hormones. The Food and Drug Administration's (FDA's) scientific measures show no distinction between the hormones naturally secreted into milk (i.e., from organically reared cows) and the additional hormones given to cows to increase milk production (i.e., conventionally reared cows).

27. Should organic foods be preferentially fed to children?

As with organic milk, there are numerous factors that go into decisions about purchasing organic fruits and vegetables. Valid scientific research comparing organically and conventionally grown foods is in its infancy, and there are little data on which to base public policy conclusions. Organic standards are set for production management and not to promote nutritional improvements in the food supply. There is some new emerging evidence that organic fruits and vegetables may have a better nutritional profile than conventionally grown foods (in the case of phytonutrients such as lycopene). How this distinction makes any difference in an individual's risk of certain diseases is far from clear.

Foods known to have the most pesticide residual on them are called the *Dirty Dozen* (actually coined by the Environmental Working Group and updated in 2011, http://www.ewg.org/foodnews) in the foodie community. They include apples, celery, strawberries, peaches, spinach, nectarines, grapes, sweet bell peppers, potatoes, blueberries, lettuce, and kale/collard greens. Those who wish to try organic foods may wish to prioritize their grocery budget by leaning towards these top 12 foods.

Additionally, foods known to have the least amount of pesticide residual on them are referred to as the *Clean 15* and they include onions, sweet corn, pineapples, avocado, asparagus, peas, mangoes, eggplant, cantaloupe, kiwi, cabbage, watermelon, sweet potatoes, grapefruit, and mushrooms. Organic varieties of these foods may not be worth the extra money to avoid pesticides.

28. Can a child get enough calcium from leafy green vegetables like spinach instead of drinking milk?

This is a trick question. Vegetables, including spinach, have a reasonable amount of calcium in them. Some vegetables, including broccoli, are a good way to get some extra calcium, and it is well absorbed. One cup of raw broccoli or a half-cup of cooked broccoli has about 30 to 40 mg of calcium. Keep this in mind when comparing calcium intakes in a child from vegetables versus an 8-ounce glass of skim milk with 300 mg of calcium in it. You must eat 10 servings of broccoli to equal the amount of calcium in one serving of milk.

Spinach is another example. One cup of raw spinach (i.e., salad greens) has about 30 mg of calcium. Cooked spinach decreases greatly in volume and concentrates the nutrients so that half a cup of cooked spinach has about 120 mg of calcium, slightly less than half the amount in a glass of milk. Also, spinach has a substance called oxalate in it that prevents the calcium from being absorbed. Oxalates in spinach are not affected much by cooking. So, virtually all of the calcium in spinach does not get absorbed very well in the body making spinach a poor choice for absorbed calcium. Milk and other dairy are the primary sources of calcium and vitamin D in our children's diet. Taking the dairy out and substituting only vegetables would make it nearly impossible to reach the RDA values for calcium and vitamin D intake without taking a supplement.

So, those who wish to avoid all milk and dairy products can get calcium and vitamin D from some vegetables, although they will need to eat many servings of these vegetables. Still, it is probably best to either use nondairy fortified food sources or supplements for children who have no dairy at all in their diet.

29. Do you get the same amount of calcium (absorbed) from soymilk as you do from cow's milk? What about almond milk?

As we noted, the best current evidence is that the amount of calcium absorbed from soymilk is about two-thirds of that from cow's milk. So, if you prefer soymilk, just drink a little more, and you will get nearly the same amount. There are no studies about almond milk that we know about, although it is likely that the results would be similar to soymilk. Almond milk is much lower in protein (1 g per 8 ounces) than either cow milk or soymilk (6 to 8 g per 8 ounces), and is often still high in added sugars. Other available products include rice milk, coconut milk, and even hemp milk. Very little testing has been done on these products to demonstrate bioavailability of calcium. Some rice milk has tricalcium phosphate as the calcium source. The bioavailability of this source is uncertain in children. In nondairy milks, calcium may precipitate out of solution and wind up at the bottom of the carton instead of in your glass. It is important to give the carton a strong, hearty shake in order to make sure the calcium stays mixed into the milk before pouring each glass.

Brands of soymilk or almond milk that are fortified with calcium and vitamin D are readily available and usually should be preferred.

30. What can you tell me about raw milk?

Raw milk is typically cow's milk that has not been pasteurized. Pasteurization is a process in which the milk is heated in order to destroy harmful bacteria. There are different types of pasteurization, but they all accomplish the same thing. Therefore, raw milk may contain harmful bacteria such as *E. coli*. Nutritionally, raw milk and pasteurized milk are the same—well—almost the same. In fact, by law pasteurized milk must have vitamin D added to it (100 IU per 8 ounces) so actually, pasteurized milk has a better nutritional profile than raw milk. Pasteurization does very little to break down the protein or lactose in milk. That is why people with cow's milk protein allergy or lactose intolerance do not have any better luck with raw milk than they do with pasteurized milk.

Some suggest that raw milk has beneficial probiotic bacteria compared to pasteurized milk. However, studies have shown that the bacteria found in raw milk are not probiotic in their biological effects. In fact, they are primarily pathogenic and may reflect poor hygiene practices during milking the animal. For good reason, we often think of yogurt as a food with probiotics. But, just because raw milk and yogurt are both dairy products, this does not mean that they both have the same healthy bacteria. Yogurt is a fermented dairy product made from milk, and during the process of making the yogurt, beneficial probiotic bacteria are added to the mixture.

31. Can you get kidney stones by drinking too much milk?

There is a condition that is currently very uncommon, called *milk alkali syndrome*, which was associated historically with very high intakes of milk, which used to be recommended for people with ulcers. The symptoms were due to high blood calcium. This condition is extremely rare nowadays.

In general, drinking milk and relatively high levels of calcium intake, at least up to the UL, are not directly associated with an increased risk of kidney stones for those not predisposed to this problem. Some well-performed studies have even shown the opposite, that a good calcium intake lowers the risk of kidney stones. There are health concerns from too much calcium, mostly related to high blood calcium and possibly calcification of arteries in the body and heart disease. It is hard for most individuals, and especially for children, to take in too much calcium from the diet.

32. Are children with celiac disease at higher risk of poor bone density?

Celiac disease is an intestinal disorder in which the body cannot tolerate a protein called *gluten*, which is commonly found in wheat, rye, and various other grains. When a child with celiac disease consumes gluten, the immune system is triggered to respond and leads to damage of the small intestine, often at the sites where calcium from the diet is absorbed into the bloodstream as it goes to the bones. With untreated or newly diagnosed celiac disease, there may be severe damage of the small intestine lining, causing malabsorption of important bone nutrients, which leads to poor bone density and increased risk of osteoporosis (http://www.niams.nih.gov/Health_Info/Bone/Osteoporosis/Conditions_Behaviors/celiac.asp).

Improved absorption of nutrients is directly related to the successful management of the disease. At this time, there are no separate recommendations for calcium or vitamin D intakes in children with celiac disease. Children whose celiac disease is well controlled will likely do well with RDA level of nutrient intake, although we encourage more research in this area. If there is concern in regard to an individual child, then a Dual-Energy X-ray Absorptiometry (DXA) scan or serum 25(OH)D may be deemed appropriate by the pediatrician.

33. I read that a group of endocrinologists has said that all Hispanic and African American children, as well as pregnant and lactating women, should get their vitamin D level tested. Is this true? What if one parent is Hispanic and the other is not? When to test in pregnancy and how often?

It is true that a group called the *Endocrine Society* made this recommendation in June 2011. See Chapter 2 for more discussion of this. This group recommended that all obese adults and children, all Hispanics, all African-Americans, and all pregnant and lactating women be tested for vitamin D deficiency. They did not specify how often or exactly when in pregnancy or lactation the testing should be done.

We do not agree with this blanket recommendation. This type of testing would involve nearly 150 million Americans and, assuming each person got several tests over a year, would cost in the $30 to $50 billion dollar range each year. All of this is recommended without the slightest proof of any benefit from such widespread testing and without consideration of the consequences to the population of this screening.

Keep an eye out for possible recommendations ultimately from other groups, such as the United States Public Health Service Task Force. Until then, we also note that the official society of obstetricians, called the *American College of Obstetrics and Gynecology* has specifically recommended that vitamin D levels are not needed routinely for pregnant women. So, this is an ongoing debate that has not been resolved yet.

Of particular concern was the suggestion by the Endocrine Society that lactating women be tested for their serum 25(OH)D. The recommendation did not indicate how often they should be tested while lactating. Since nonlactating women who are formula-feeding are not recommended for routine testing by this group, the implication is that an extra burden of blood testing would be put on women who choose to breast-feed their infants. This burden is based on concern, not supported by evidence reviewed by other groups, including the IOM, that lactation would be a risk to maternal health without high vitamin D levels.

Regardless, the effects on lactation could be substantial. Currently, there are no routine blood or other medical tests recommended specifically for women who are breast-feeding. Adding such a recommendation would not be consistent with efforts to increase breast-feeding without a strong reason to perform such testing, which we do not believe exists.

34. Why shouldn't everyone just take the upper level amounts of vitamin D, which, after all, the IOM said were safe intakes? Some people are told to do this with the claim that this is the recommendation of all experts in this field.

The upper limits are not intended to be a *usual intake* for healthy individuals. They are developed based on looking at the lowest intake that led to some evidence of toxicity or the highest intake that did not show any toxicity. Most of the time, however, the exact amount of these nutrients that causes a side effect simply is not known. Furthermore, there is a huge interindividual variation in how much does cause a problem. Finally, even if we can estimate, based on some experience, how much is a toxic intake, rarely, if ever, do we know if that same amount would be more or less harmful over a long period of time (e.g., decades).

Therefore, the upper limits, such as those for calcium and vitamin D, involve a substantial amount of uncertainty. This is especially true for the upper level values in children where usually we have almost no real data for long-term risks.

The EAR and RDAs are based on evidence of benefit. They are amounts that are considered both safe and likely to be effective in maintaining health. As one moves up from the RDA to the UL, the risks of toxicity begin to develop, the uncertainty of benefit increases, and the unknown aspects of long-term consequences increases.

Specific to vitamin D, the short-term safety margin is probably fairly large for intakes between the RDA and the UL, and it is very unlikely that most children, especially those after the first year of age, would suffer any toxic effects from long-term intakes around the UL values. However, there is uncertainty in this, and there is no reason to take in high doses of any nutrient until there is more evidence of long-term benefit. Arguments that high-dose supplements are equivalent to usual or ancient sunshine exposure are not grounded in modern science and do not represent a reason to use high-dose vitamin D supplements.

Finally, one needs to be cautious about nutrient interactions when taking high doses. If one takes the UL for calcium and vitamin D, and the UL for every other vitamin and mineral, then it can be difficult to know if there may be some problems with the relative intakes of these minerals affecting other mineral bioavailability. Based on current dietary patterns, individuals do not reach the upper level of calcium or vitamin D very often from diet, only from diet combined with relatively high-dose supplements. There is not a lot of long-term evidence about the safety of high-dose, multinutrient supplement use, especially in children.

35. Is high-fructose corn syrup bad for children?

We have no idea. Really, we have made it to the end of this book and avoided all controversy (well, not exactly). Why take on a tough issue like this now? A more serious answer is that like everything, moderation is the key. There is a fairly strong body of evidence that high-fructose corn syrup is somewhat worse metabolically than normal sugar, but the evidence, in our opinion, is not as overwhelming as is sometimes portrayed, especially if the high-fructose corn syrup–containing food or beverage is limited to an occasional serving. Children who are overweight probably should be more cautious in their intake of high-fructose corn syrup.

36. Did Mozart die of vitamin D deficiency?

A recent letter to the editor of a medical journal received a good bit of publicity as it claimed that a likely cause of Mozart's untimely and youthful demise was vitamin D deficiency. It was claimed this exacerbated his well-known pulmonary problems and was worsened by the large percentage of time he spent indoors and the likely limited sunshine exposure he had. Remarkably, this story got a lot of attention on the Internet, and in blogs and news articles. Many headlined their article with things such as, "Mozart Probably Died Young from Not Getting Enough Sun." (http://www.businessinsider.com/ mozart-died-35-not-enough-sun-2011-7).*

It is impossible to draw a serum 25(OH)D on Mozart now to know if he was deficient. Even if the serum was low, there is no proof that this was related to whatever chronic disorders he had that led to his death. Therefore, it is impossible to argue this issue in a meaningful way. The real question is, why, absent any evidence that respiratory diseases in adults during Mozart's era were vitamin D-related, did this get such publicity and were people ready to believe this assertion without any evidence? There are lots of people even now with very low serum 25(OH)D levels, and although not all are healthy, they are not routinely dying of respiratory diseases even in countries with limited sanitation and antibiotics. Those who believe that vitamin D deficiency causes almost all human diseases are enthused by such speculation about Mozart.

Other people wonder why anyone thought that there was any meaningful evidence that Mozart's demise was related to any nutritional disorder? It would be more intellectually honest to simply say that one believes poor sanitation, hygiene, and so forth, in the 18th century was exacerbated by inadequate sunshine and low vitamin D levels causing increased morbidity. That would be a bit harder to quote in the media though. It might even be true, although it would always just be a hypothesis.

We have no idea why Mozart died. Neither does anyone else.

For those who are Harry Potter fans, we offer up the following dubious analogy for consideration. We have been concerned about the tendency of Slytherin house members to live underground on the effects of vitamin D status, as noted in the second book of the series, *Harry Potter and the Chamber of Secrets*. "The Slytherin common room is a long, low underground room (strategically located under the Hogwarts lake)." Lack of vitamin D from spending so much time underground might be a big part of their antisocial tendencies. Perhaps this time underground and the vitamin D deficiency led to the development of evil *death eaters*? Who knows? Hard to imagine what else could be responsible! Salazar Slytherin might have died from vitamin D deficiency? Only J.K. Rowling knows for certain.

---

* Grant WB, Pilz S, 2011, Vitamin D Deficiency Contributed to Mozart's Death, *Med Probl Perform Art* 26(2):117.

37. What is the difference between vitamin D_2 and vitamin D_3 and how should this affect how vitamin D supplements are selected?

This is an extremely common question. Vitamin D that is naturally made via skin conversion is vitamin D_3. Vitamin D_3 is also called *cholecalciferol* and vitamin D_2 is called *ergocalciferol*. Foods may be fortified with either vitamin D_2 or vitamin D_3. We will defer a detailed chemical description of the differences and focus on the functional ones. Vitamin D_3 is the form naturally made from sunshine exposure. Numerous studies have compared both forms related to biological outcomes. Unfortunately, the results of these studies have been mixed. However, the general consensus is that vitamin D_3 is both more active and safer than vitamin D_2, although this difference is probably magnified at higher doses. Regardless, it is generally best to purchase supplements of vitamin D_3, whenever possible.

38. Dr. Abrams, if you could reconsider the dietary reference intakes (DRIs) now (late 2011), based on what has been discussed and published since they were released at the end of November 2010, would you recommend changing anything?

I have had the chance to review a huge amount of literature related to calcium and vitamin D requirements that has been released since the IOM report of November 2010, which was finalized several months before then. On the whole, related specifically to pediatrics, pregnancy, and lactation, the only thing, based on new information, that I would consider recommending be changed is increasing the RDA for vitamin D in adolescents from 600 IU to 800 IU per day. This is based on some recent findings since the IOM report was released suggesting the higher intake might more reliably achieve serum levels of 25(OH)D in teenagers at or above 20 ng/mL. This is a relatively minor change, and it is far from certain that this is needed.

I have no opinion about reconsidering any of the 2011 DRI values for healthy nonpregnant, nonlactating adults, although some of these have been vigorously debated since the IOM report was released. I do not personally expect the DRI report on calcium and vitamin D to be revisited by the IOM in the next 10 to 15 years. There are many other compelling nutritional issues that the IOM needs to evaluate through this process before returning again to these. I am certain that having done it twice, I have no intent on being on such a panel for a third time. The evidence base will need to develop during the next decade or more before these issues are revisited. The ongoing controlled trial of vitamin D and omega-3 supplementation in adults conducted by Dr. Manson from the Harvard School of Public Health may be a key piece of the future data we have. In all probability, we will not have similar data from a population of children and will continue to have to make use of physiological studies and association studies. Hopefully, a few controlled clinical trials will be conducted, however.

Index